# Congenital Toxoplasmosis in Humans and Domestic Animals

## Edited by

### Katia Denise Saraiva Bresciani

*UNESP, Universidade Estadual Paulista Júlio de Mesquita Filho (Unesp)*
*Faculdade de Medicina Veterinária de Araçatuba Araçatuba, São Paulo*
*Brasil*


### Alvimar José da Costa

*UNESP, Universidade Estadual Paulista Júlio de Mesquita Filho (Unesp)*
*Faculdade de Ciências Agrárias e Veterinárias de Jaboticabal,*
*CPPAR Centro de Pesquisas em Sanidade Animal*
*Jaboticabal, São Paulo Brasil*

## General:

1. Any dispute or claim arising out of or in connection with this License Agreement or the Work (including non-contractual disputes or claims) will be governed by and construed in accordance with the laws of the U.A.E. as applied in the Emirate of Dubai. Each party agrees that the courts of the Emirate of Dubai shall have exclusive jurisdiction to settle any dispute or claim arising out of or in connection with this License Agreement or the Work (including non-contractual disputes or claims).
2. Your rights under this License Agreement will automatically terminate without notice and without the need for a court order if at any point you breach any terms of this License Agreement. In no event will any delay or failure by Bentham Science Publishers in enforcing your compliance with this License Agreement constitute a waiver of any of its rights.
3. You acknowledge that you have read this License Agreement, and agree to be bound by its terms and conditions. To the extent that any other terms and conditions presented on any website of Bentham Science Publishers conflict with, or are inconsistent with, the terms and conditions set out in this License Agreement, you acknowledge that the terms and conditions set out in this License Agreement shall prevail.

**Bentham Science Publishers Ltd.**
Executive Suite Y - 2
PO Box 7917, Saif Zone
Sharjah, U.A.E.
Email: subscriptions@benthamscience.org

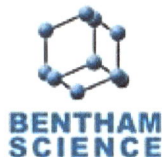

**BENTHAM
SCIENCE**

# CONTENTS

# FOREWORD

Toxoplasmosis is a disease that has, as its etiologic agent, the protozoa *Toxoplasma gondii*. The disease is of cosmopolitan occurrence, being prevalent in humans and animals, with infection rates that vary with the geographical region, attaining 70-80% in some ecosystems, in different herds and human populations, with infection in most cases being unapparent.

Despite the importance of clinical toxoplasmosis in adults, with a wider variety of clinical signs and symptoms, due to the species affected and/or the strain of the parasite involved, the issue that is most delicate, and of greatest preoccupation, is gestational and congenital toxoplasmosis.

Since generally, this is a silent infection in the prospective mother or pregnant females, this preoccupation extends from the difficulty to diagnose maternal and fetal infections, including the few existing methods for fetal diagnosis, where most of these are invasive and frequently place the fetus at risk.

The objective of this book is not to establish a parallel between congenital infections in the different species, but to demonstrate the implications, damages and losses for each female considering the individual and collective aspects.

This book clearly describes and demonstrates the sanitary impacts of toxoplasmosis in the fetal impairment, during gestation via transplacental transmission, with impact on livestock, which can result in elevated losses to animal production, as well as on companion animals, where the loss of young animals affects emotionally the families involved. In addition, in humans, where the sequels and clinical signs, even retarded, are extremely serious, principally when there are neurological and ocular signs.

Based on the best scientific studies available, the authors have used their vast professional experience to demonstrate procedures, including those related to the aspects of management of toxoplasmosis that are still controversial in females from several species, as well as gestating and lactating mothers, using a realistic approach.

This publication is particularly timely at the moment when toxoplasmosis has been recognized as an important problem in humans and animals, when there is need for One Health, during which human health is directly related to animal health and the environment, and vice versa.

Whenever we write books, publish articles or present a paper, we must have in our minds, as clearly as possible, the affirmation of Carlyle Guerra de Macedo, who was the Director of Pan American Health Organization, relative to the responsibility of what is being published: "It must be remembered that behind each table, every report or every material examined, there are lives, there are people, there is suffering, waiting for our efforts and human solidarity".

Above all, this book has this concern and responsibility. The chapters within this book are **not only a collection of technical information acquired from existing literature, but are** additionally, the results of years of work of the team involved with patients and communities.

Many of these have served to evaluate procedures and conducts as well as to experience orientations and formed the basis of this publication. Consequently, we have the expectation to demonstrate that each chapter was also written by the hands of patients and their communities, so that these are the main actors and authors of this book.

**Italmar T. Navarro**
Centro de Ciências Agrárias
Universidade Estadual de Londrina
Paraná
Brazil

# PREFACE

This book focuses on the epidemiology, pathogenesis, clinical aspects, prevention and control of congenital *Toxoplasma gondii* infections in humans and domestic animals (pets and livestock). Toxoplasmosis is a zoonotic disease. In humans, it is essential to aim for implementation of control programs, including preventive measures that promotes early diagnosis and appropriate indication of adequate antiparasitic treatments to pregnant women, being therefore able to diminish the seriousness of sequelae of toxoplasmosis in fetuses. Important aspects for control programs of congenital toxoplasmosis, and for maternal and neonatal screening of toxoplasmosis control programs, were reviewed. Additionally, based on this information, reproductive disorders such as abortion, neonatal mortality and prematurity due to infection by *Toxoplasma gondii*, may be more easily diagnosed by veterinarians, of both small and large animals medical clinics, in their routine daily care. Under the zoonotic aspect, health professionals may become aware of these clinical signs and take preventive measures for their control.

The book **"Congenital Toxoplasmosis in Human and Domestic Animals"** is a compilation of eight chapters, contributions of established researchers in the field, with content directed to the study of epidemiology, pathogenesis, clinical aspects and control of congenital *T. gondii* infections in humans and domestic animals (pets and production).

In the first chapter, Dr. Ragozo has shed some light on the parasite, its life cycle, clinical signs, diagnosis and some epidemiological aspects of toxoplasmosis.

In the second chapter, Dr. Navarro and his colleagues discuss the epidemiology and impact of human congenital toxoplasmosis, pathogenesis, genotypic characterization, diagnosis, therapy, prevention and control.

Then, in the third chapter, Dr. Camossi and collaborators discuss reproductive problems on female dogs and emphasize the attention, which should be paid regarding occurrence of this parasite in canine populations.

In the fourth chapter, Dr. Galvão and colleagues describe the main manifestations, prevention and treatment of congenital toxoplasmosis in cats.

In the fifth chapter, Dr. Lopes and collaborators discuss the different reproductive alterations in sheep with toxoplasmosis and reinforce the possibility of sexual transmission of *T. gondii* in this animal species. The same authors, in the sixth chapter, demonstrate that congenital transmission of this disease in goats can result in disorders in the offspring (regardless of pregnancy stage), which can subsequently lead to severe losses or prejudice to descendants and their owners.

In the seventh chapter, Dr. Garcia discusses aspects related to parasite-host relationship between *T. gondii* and pigs, such as epidemiology, natural infection (congenital) and experimental infections, diagnosis, vaccines and prevention.

Finally, in the eighth chapter, Dr. Santos and colleagues describe the various aspects of congenital form and the importance of cattle on the epidemiology of toxoplasmosis.

The publication of this book would not have been possible without the sincere efforts of the authors of each chapter, and especially the staff at Bentham Science Publishers, giving their continuous support. Perhaps, of greater importance than the book and its many contributions, were the remarkable people that formed a unique collaborative team to make it happen.

**Katia Denise Saraiva Bresciani**
Faculdade de Medicina Veterinária de Araçatuba
Unesp, Universidade Estadual Paulista
Araçatuba
Brasil

**Alvimar José da Costa**
Faculdade de Ciências Agrárias e Veterinárias de Jaboticabal
Unesp, Universidade Estadual Paulista
Jaboticabal
Brasil

# DEDICATION

*Thanks*
*To God, for all blessings in every morning...*
And to all the people who somehow find themselves in our lines...

# SUMMARY

This book is of outstanding interest to epidemiologists, doctors, veterinarians and public health specialists. Important aspects for control programs of congenital toxoplasmosis and for maternal and neonatal screening of toxoplasmosis control programs were discussed. Additionally, based on this information, reproductive disorders such as abortion, neonatal mortality and prematurity due to infection by *Toxoplasma gondii*, maybe more easily diagnosed in their routine daily care. Under the zoonotic aspect, health professionals may become aware of these clinical signs and take preventive measures for their control.

# List of Contributors

| | |
|---|---|
| **Alessandra Mara Alves Ragozo** | Universidade Estadual Paulista (Unesp), Instituto de Biociências de Botucatu, Botucatu, São Paulo, Brasil |
| **André Luiz Baptista Galvão** | Universidade Estadual Paulista (Unesp), Faculdade de Ciências Agrárias e Veterinárias, Jaboticabal, São Paulo, Brasil<br>UNIRP, Centro Universitário de Rio Preto, Faculdade de Medicina Veterinária, São José do Rio Preto, São Paulo, Brasil |
| **Breno Cayeiro Cruz** | Universidade Estadual Paulista (Unesp), Centro de Pesquisas em Sanidade Animal Faculdade de Ciências Agrárias e Veterinárias, Jaboticabal, São Paulo, Brasil |
| **Celso Tetsuo Nagase Suzuki** | Instituto de Computação (Laboratory of Image Data Science/LIDS), Universidade Estadual de Campinas (Unicamp), São Paulo, Brasil |
| **Daniel Fontana Ferreira Cardia** | UNICAMP, Universidade Estadual de Campinas, Instituto de Computação, Campinas, São Paulo, Brasil |
| **Edna Maria Vissoci Reiche** | UEL, Universidade Estadual de Londrina Professor, Departamento of Patologia, Análises Clínicas e Toxicológicas Centro de Ciências da Saúde, Londrina, Paraná, Brasil |
| **Fabiana Maria Ruiz Lopes Mori** | Unifil, Centro Universitário Filadélfia, Centro de Ciências Saúde, Londrina, Paraná, Brasil |
| **Italmar Teodorico Navarro** | UEL, Universidade Estadual de Londrina Professor, Departamento of Medicina Veterinária Preventiva Centro de Ciências Agrárias, Londrina, Paraná, Brasil |
| **Inacio Teruo Inoue** | UEL, Universidade Estadual de Londrina, Departamento of Ginecologia e Obstetrícia Centro de Ciências da Saúde, Londrina, Paraná, Brasil |
| **Jancarlo Ferreira Gomes** | Instituto de Computação (Laboratory of Image Data Science/LIDS), Faculdade de Ciências Médicas and Universidade Estadual de Campinas (Unicamp), São Paulo, Brasil |
| **Jaqueline Dario Capobiango** | UEL, Universidade Estadual de Londrina Professor, Departamento of Pediatria e Cirurgia Pediátrica Centro de Ciências da Saúde, Londrina, Paraná, Brasil |
| **João Luis Garcia** | UEL, Universidade Estadual de Londrina, Departamento of Medicina Veterinária Preventiva, Laboratório de Protozoologia Centro de Ciências Agrárias, Londrina, Paraná, Brasil |
| **Lucilene Granuzzio Camossi** | UNICAMP, Universidade Estadual de Campinas, Instituto de Computação, Campinas, São Paulo, Brasil |
| **Maerle Oliveira Maia** | Unir, Fundaçãp Universidade Federal de Rondônia, Departamento de Medicina Veterinária, Brasil |
| **Regina Mitsuka-Breganó** | UEL, Universidade Estadual de Londrina, Departamento of Medicina Veterinária Preventiva Centro de Ciências Agrárias, Londrina, Paraná, Brasil |

**Selwyn Arligton Headley**    UEL, Universidade Estadual de Londrina, Departamento of Medicina Veterinária Preventiva Centro de Ciências Agrárias, Londrina, Paraná, Brasil

**Thaís Rabelo dos Santos**    Universidade Federal dos Vales do Jequitinhonha e Mucuri, Campus Unaí Instituto de Ciências Agrárias, Minas Gerais, Brasil

**Victor José Vieira Rosseto**    Professor, UNIRP, Centro Universitário de Rio Preto, Faculdade de Medicina Veterinária, São José do Rio Preto, São Paulo, Brasil

**Welber Daniel Zanetti Lopes**    UFG, Universidade Federal de Goiás, Regional de Jataí, Brasil

**Weslen Fabricio Pires Teixeira**    Researcher, UNESP, Universidade Estadual Paulista Julio de Mesquita Filho, Campus de Araçatuba, Brasil

# CHAPTER 1

# *Toxoplasma gondii*

## Alessandra M.A. Ragozo[1,*]

[1] *Departamento de Parasitologia, Universidade Estadual Paulista (Unesp), Instituto de Biociências, Botucatu, São Paulo, Brasil*

**Abstract:** *Toxoplasma gondii* is an obligate intracellular parasite, and its infectious stages are: sporozoites, tachyzoites and bradyzoites in tissue cysts. The life cycle of *T. gondii* is a heteroxenous system that alternates between sexual and asexual stages. Ingestion of raw or undercooked meat with cysts, sporulated oocysts and congenital infections is the principal route of infection. *T. gondii* usually parasitizes the host without producing clinical signs. However, the infection leads to several neurological and ocular problems, and lead immunosuppressed individuals to severe clinical conditions. For livestock animals, the infection leads to abortion and neonate mortality. The prevalence of antibodies is reported worldwide in humans and animals. Toxoplasmosis is considered one of the most important parasitic infections of human. For diagnosis and epidemiologic studies, several methods are used, for instance: serology to detect antibodies anti-*T.gondii*, parasite isolation in laboratory animals (bioassays) or protozoan observation through direct molecular methods to detect the DNA of *T. gondii*. Recent studies on *T. gondii* virulence and genotyping using standard methods revealed different results in South America, Africa and Asia. These results were different from those observed in North America and Europe.

**Keywords:** Apicomplexa, Bioassays, Coccidian parasite, Diagnosis, Epidemiology, Genotyping, Isolate, Isolation, Life cycle, Molecular epidemiology, Protozoan, PCR-RFLP, q_PCR, Serology, Toxoplasmosis, Virulence, Zoonosis.

## INTRODUCTION

Toxoplasmosis is a cosmopolitan zoonosis, caused by *Toxoplasma gondii,* an obligate intracellular parasite, infecting virtually any mammal and bird species [1]. Due to its medical and veterinary importance, this parasite has been intensely studied among the coccidia. However, several aspects of the biology, epidemiology and molecular methods are still being investigated [2, 3].

* **Corresponding author Alessandra M. Ragozo:** Departamento de Parasitologia, Universidade Estadual Paulista (Unesp), Instituto de Biociências, Botucatu, São Paulo, Brazil; Tel/Fax: 05514 3880 0522; E-mail: aleragozo@ibb.unesp.b

The first description of this protozoan was carried out in France by Nicolle and Manceux, in 1908, in a wild rodent (*Ctenodactylus gundi*). Simultaneously, Splendore described it in rabbits in Brazil. The term *Toxoplasma* comes from the Greek and refers to its shape resembling a rising bow (toxon = bow; plasma = shape), and the word *gondii* refers to the rodent in which it was first described. In 1909, the genus *Toxoplasma* was introduced in the phylum Apicomplexa [1].

The most important transmission routes of this protozoan are transplacental transmission, ingestion of meat infected with tissue cysts, and the ingestion of food and water contaminated with sporulated oocysts [1, 3, 4]. Considering that one of the transmission routes of *T. gondii* is by the consumption of raw or undercooked meat and even unpasteurized milk, infected animals may represent an infection source for humans and for other species of carnivorous animals [5 - 7].

*T. gondii* can be found in three basic morphological forms: tachyzoites, fast replication forms are characteristic in the acute phase of infection; bradyzoites, slow replication forms, observed in tissue cysts in the chronic or latent phase of infection; and sporozoites, present in the oocysts that are eliminated in the feces of infected felids [1].

Tachyzoites are approximately 5 µm long and 2 µm wide, possess a pointed anterior part and rounded posterior part, with the nucleus in the middle part. The apical complex is located in the anterior area and is composed by polar and apical rings, conoid, rhoptries and micronemes. The apical complex is involved in the host cell invasion and formation of the parasitophorus vacuole.

The nucleus is located at the central area and the Golgi complex is located above. Elements of the endoplasmic reticulum and branched mitochondria are present in the interior of the nucleus envelope. The acidocalcisomes, dense granules and amylopectin granules are present in variable numbers and locations [8]. The external membranes and cytoskeleton are involved in the integrity and motility of the tachyzoites [1, 3].

Bradyzoites result from the conversion of tachyzoites into a latent metabolism and characterize the chronic phase of the disease, forming tissue cysts with variable shapes: in brain cells, they are rounded while in muscle cells they are ellipsoid, ranging in size from 10 µm in young cysts to 100 µm in old cysts [3]. The cyst wall has a thickness of up to 0.5 µm, enveloping hundreds of bradyzoites. The cysts may be infectious in carcasses refrigerated from 1 to 6 °C, however, the freezing process inactivates the viability of the cysts when in -12 °C for 3 days [3] and when cooking at 67 °C degrees [9].

Sporozoites are infective forms observed inside mature oocysts. Oocysts excreted from cats are non-sporulated subspherical to spherical shape and measure approximately 10 to 12 μm of diameter; the cyst wall of the oocyst is composed of two layers without polar granules. The sporulation process occurs from one to five days after being eliminated and oocysts sub-hemispheric to ellipsoid in shape, developing two sporocysts containing, each, four sporozoites [1]. Mature oocysts are resistant to disinfectants and, under warm and humid environmental conditions can survive for longer periods. However, they are inactivated by freezing at minus 6 to 7 °C degrees or when exposed to 37 °C for one day [3, 10].

## LIFE CYCLE

Life cycle of *T. gondii* is heteroxenous and the transmission of the parasite from host to host is associated with alimentary habits involving a predator-prey system that alternates between definitive hosts [sexual stage] and intermediate hosts [asexual stage].

The multiplication occurs under the forms tachyzoites and bradyzoites, although the sexual stage of development occurs only in the definitive hosts, the felids (domestic and wild cats).

Felids (domestic and wild cats) are the definitive hosts and are infected after ingestion of tissues from intermediate hosts harboring cysts. During the digestion process the cyst wall is destroyed by gastric enzymes and the bradyzoites are released in the intestinal tract. The parasite actively invades the epithelial cells in the small intestine starting sequential stages of asexual multiplications and the development of schizonts with merozoites [1 - 3].

The sexual multiplication occurs after the enteroepithelial development and differentiation of male and female gametes (gametogony). After fertilization, the oocysts are formed and eliminated in the feces of infected felids, contaminating the environment. Oocysts excretion can be detected from three to seven days after ingestion of the cysts and can last for more than 20 days. During this period cats can eliminate approximately 100 million oocysts, that will become infectious in the environment after five to seven days depending on humidity and temperature conditions [1, 3, 11].

Intermediate hosts can be infected after ingestion of sporulated oocysts contaminating food and water sources. The sporozoites are released during the digestion process and penetrate the intestinal epithelium where they differentiate into tachyzoites. Tachyzoites are rapidly multiplying forms and actively invade and replicate inside any nucleated cell. After seven to ten days of infection, the conversion of tachyzoites to bradyzoites can be observed forming tissue cysts located predominantly in the muscle and brain [1, 3].

Another route of infection is by ingestion of raw or undercooked meat with tissue cysts. Bradyzoites are released after gastric digestion and can remain viable for one to two hours after the cyst wall disruption. After penetrating the intestinal epithelium, the bradizoites rapidly return to tachyzoite stage and initiates the invasion of host cells [3].

Regardless of the infection route, congenital toxoplasmosis or secondary infection is observed when the acute phase of the infection occurs during pregnancy, in which the parasite is transmitted to the fetus through the placenta. Tachyzoites present in the maternal blood cross the placenta and infect the fetus [1, 3].

## CLINICAL SIGNS

*T. gondii* is an opportunistic parasite and usually does not produce severe symptoms in immunocompetent hosts. Chronic infections lead to the formation of latent cysts that may last throughout the host's life.

The major clinical condition of toxoplasmosis refers to (a) primary infection during pregnancy, which may result in congenital infection of the fetus, causing several neurological and ocular problems, such as intellectual disabilities and blindness, abortion and neonate mortality; and (b) reactivation of latent infections in immunosuppressed individuals, which leads to severe clinical conditions, sometimes lethal [1, 2].

Toxoplasmosis is often presented as asymptomatic in most of the hosts, however fever, cervical lymphadenopathy or other nonspecific clinical sign could be observed in immunocompetent individuals [12 - 14]. Abortion or congenital alterations like hydrocephaly, cerebral calcification, intellectual disability and ocular toxoplasmosis are clinical observations in the congenital transmission of *T. gondii* [15, 16]. It must be highlighted that the age factor, host species, virulence of the parasite, infectious dosage and infection route can influence the development of the infection [1, 15, 17].

## DIAGNOSIS

Diagnosis of *T. gondii* infection is made using laboratory methods associated to clinical and epidemiological data. Early identification and treatment can reduce the congenital transmission and consequences of *T. gondii* infection in newborns and immunodeficient patients.

There are several serological techniques to detect specific antibody responses like the Dye Test (DT), Indirect Haemagglutination (IHA), and Complement Fixation

(CF). However, the most commonly used tests are Indirect Fluorescent Antibody Test (IFAT), Modified Agglutination Test (MAT), and Enzyme-Linked Immunosorbent Assay (ELISA) [2, 20]. The combination of serological tests enables to determine whether the infection is chronic or recently acquired [1, 15]. For pregnant women, it is indicated that the serological screening to diagnose infection during pregnancy, in order to detect cases of acute infection or monitor seronegative pregnant women [17]. The serological tests are also used in epidemiological studies to detect antibodies, aiming to determine the occurrence of the agent in the population and in livestock herds [2, 21 - 23].

For *T. gondii* identification in cat feces, specific *T. gondii* polymerase chain reaction (PCR) is recommended for confirmation and differential diagnosis from *Hammondia hammondi* oocysts. Sensitivity of faecal exams can be increased by using flotation techniques [24].

*T. gondii* isolation from clinical or food samples can be obtained by inoculation in laboratory animals and cell cultures. Inoculation in mice enables to evaluate the infectivity and compare virulence between isolates [1, 21, 25], which is measured by the disease evolution, morbidity and mortality rate. Biological characterization of different *T. gondii* isolates were determined based on their virulence in mice and have led to the classification of highly virulent, non-virulent or of intermediate virulence [1].

Molecular methods are used to detect the DNA of *T. gondii* in a wide variety of clinical samples from animals and humans worldwide [26]. DNA amplification and molecular characterization are also used for epidemiological studies, detecting the occurrence of distinct genotypes of the agent [21, 25, 27, 28]. Molecular methods can be divided into two groups: one includes techniques used for specific detection of *T. gondii* DNA in biological samples, as quantitative real time PCR [*q*PCR]; and the second group involves molecular techniques of high resolution to identify isolates of the agent, such as *multilocus* PCR-RFLP, microsatellite analyses, and *multilocus* sequence typing (MLST) [26].

## EPIDEMIOLOGY

Toxoplasmosis is considered one of the most important parasitic infections in humans. Its occurrence is cosmopolitan and the prevalence varies among populations. In the USA, an occurrence of approximately 30% of the population is estimated [13], and in some countries of Central Europe the values range from 37 to 58% of seropositive children and pregnant women [2]. In Brazil, the prevalence is higher, ranging from 21.5 [29] to 97.4% [30]. The difference observed in serum antibody prevalence among ethnic groups is closely related to environmental and socio-cultural aspects, like feeding habits and sanitary conditions, which is reflected in the epidemiology of *T. gondii* [2].

Toxoplasmosis outbreaks in humans are generally reported in small groups of individuals or families [2, 31 - 33], but it can also involve a greater number of infected people [14]. Most of the times, outbreaks may be related to virulent strain that determine clinical signs and characterize toxoplasmic infection [14, 34]. The occurrence of outbreaks of *T. gondii* infection is also observed in livestock; however these are less reported due to the lack of visible symptoms or even confused with other diseases [35].

Due to cultural and feeding habits, toxoplasmosis outbreaks identified in human beings have shown that the source of infection varies among populations, and can occur by ingestion of raw meat with tissue cysts of *T. gondii* [32, 36, 37], consumption of water and food contaminated with oocysts [14, 38, 39], ingestion of unpasteurized milk of infected animals [40], and outbreaks of congenital toxoplasmosis where pregnant women have the habit of eating jerked beef, seal liver and raw meat of caribou [31].

Prevalence of anti-*T.gondii* antibodies is reported worldwide in several domestic, livestock, and wild animals [1]. In Brazil, seroepidemiological surveys in animals demonstrated the dissemination of the protozoan throughout the country [22] revealing high seroprevalence, with values close to 90% for some swine and caprine populations, 75% for capybaras, 59% for ovine and 49% for bovines [22]. Besides seroprevalence studies, isolations of viable *T. gondii* cysts were obtained in bioassays carried out with tissue samples of seropositive animals from slaughterhouses, therefore those animals are possible source of infection for the population [21, 41 - 43].

Despite the high seroprevalence observed in bovine herds [44] isolates *T. gondii* in only six out of 16 dams detected as positive in the bioassay had antibody titers to *T. gondii* detected by IFAT. There is an established correlation between anti-*T. gondii* antibodies and tissue cysts in sheep [45], however, this has not been found in cattle [46]. Nevertheless, experimental studies demonstrated that positive serology results in bovine are not a good indicator of viable tissue cysts [47]. Another relevant aspect is the selection of tissue samples, since *T. gondii* can be detected in several tissues of bovines, apparently presenting no predilection sites for the establishment of this parasite, as in swine, where viable cysts are usually detected in diaphragm and heart muscle tissues [47].

Generally, caprine, ovine and swine are more sensitive to infection when compared to bovines, equines and poultry, in which toxoplasmosis are rarely observed [2]. It should be noted that clinical manifestation of toxoplasmosis in animals, as well as in humans, depends mainly on the species susceptibility, host immune response and virulence of the *T. gondii* isolate [1, 15].

Regarding virulence, there is considerable variability in the different isolates of *T. gondii,* either from human or animal origin. The mouse *Mus musculus* is the main laboratory animal used as experimental model for toxoplasmosis and, through bioassays in this species, has resulted in several studies of virulence characterization during isolation of the agent [18, 21, 25, 41, 42, 48].

Despite several factors influence the virulence of *T. gondii*, including route of inoculation, the parasite stage, animal species and parasite genotype [3, 49], there have been studies associating virulence in mice [phenotype] with the parasite genotype, demonstrating heterogeneity of biological behavior of different isolates of the agent, suggesting existence of high DNA polymorphism, which influences the pathogenicity of *T. gondii* infection [50, 51].

There have been intense studies associating the severity of the disease in humans and animals to the initial virulence of the sample. The virulence of *T. gondii* isolates is used to be based on observations obtained from bioassays in mice, however, with the development of genetic markers, it is possible now to detect genotypic variability among isolates of humans and animals [1, 22].

Even differing in some biological properties, possibility of genetic recombination in its definitive host, and with worldwide distribution; initial studies of *T. gondii* genotyping [3, 12, 51] revealed that *T. gondii* isolates were antigenic and morphologically similar in its capacity of infecting a variety of hosts and still exhibiting low genetic variation [3, 12, 50], suggesting a clonal population structure [51]. However, such information was obtained from isolates in Europe and North America, which were grouped in three genotypes: Type I, II and III [51].

Studies on *T. gondii* genotyping have started over 20 years ago, by isoenzymatic analyses, or by restriction fragment length polymorphism (RFLP) generated by restriction enzymes. After that, the use of microsatellite analyses [52 - 54] and new markers in the PCR-RFLP [25, 26, 55, 56], allowed more detailed studies of *T. gondii* genotyping.

There have been reports of genotyping and virulence of *T. gondii* since 2002, exhibiting divergent results from the ones obtained before [21, 41 - 43]. Different results were also observed in other countries in South America, Africa and Asia [3], revealing a complex populational structure with high level of genotypic variability, indicating the existence of recombinant lineages [57, 58].

According to Su *et al.* [55], the standardization of markers used in *T. gondii* genotyping enables comparisons of genotyping and biological attributes of the parasite, allowing to group the genotypes observed all over the world and the description of haplogroups. Some of these haplogroups are widely distributed along the continents when considering clonal lineages [3, 59]. However, there are atypical samples that remain isolated with single polymorphism and cannot be grouped in any of the haplogroups [3, 59]. To date, besides the three lineages initially described [types I, II and III], 12 haplogroups have been described, but these haplogroups are not totally homogeneous, the use of more specific markers being necessary to refine and enable a sub grouping that may be associated with the geographical origin and phenotypic characteristic [3, 60].

Considering the strong zoonotic potential of toxoplasmosis, the investigation of genotypes from animal infections and from products of animal origin may be of great informative importance, either for verifying the correlation between strain type found and biological properties, or for epidemiological tracking of the agent in order to identify sources of infection or transmission routes [61].

## CONSENT FOR PUBLICATION

Not applicable.

## CONFLICT OF INTEREST

The authors declare no conflict of interest, financial or otherwise.

## ACKNOWLEDGEMENTS

Declared none.

## REFERENCES

[1]     Dubey JP. Toxoplasmosis of animals and humans. 2a ed. Boca Raton: CRC Press; 2010.

[2]     Tenter AM, Heckeroth AR, Weiss LM. *Toxoplasma gondii*: from animals to humans. Int J Parasitol 2000; 30(12-13): 1217-58.
[http://dx.doi.org/10.1016/S0020-7519(00)00124-7] [PMID: 11113252]

[3]     Robert-Gangneux F, Dardé ML. Epidemiology of and diagnostic strategies for toxoplasmosis. Clin Microbiol Rev 2012; 25(2): 264-96.
[http://dx.doi.org/10.1128/CMR.05013-11] [PMID: 22491772]

[4]     Dubey JP. Oocyst shedding by cats fed isolated bradyzoites and comparison of infectivity of bradyzoites of the VEG strain *Toxoplasma gondii* to cats and mice. J Parasitol 2001; 87(1): 215-9.
[http://dx.doi.org/10.1645/0022-3395(2001)087[0215:OSBCFI]2.0.CO;2] [PMID: 11227895]

[5]     Vitor RW, Pinto JB, Chiari CD. Eliminação de *Toxoplasma gondii* através de urina, saliva e leite de caprinos experimentalmente infectados. Arq Bras Med Vet Zootec 1991; 43(2): 147-54.

[6]     Dubey JP, Verma SK, Ferreira LR, *et al.* Detection and survival of *Toxoplasma gondii* in milk and cheese from experimentally infected goats. J Food Prot 2014; 77(10): 1747-53.

[http://dx.doi.org/10.4315/0362-028X.JFP-14-167] [PMID: 25285492]

[7]     da Silva JG, Alves BH, Melo RP, *et al.* Occurrence of anti-*Toxoplasma gondii* antibodies and parasite DNA in raw milk of sheep and goats of local breeds reared in Northeastern Brazil. Acta Trop 2015; 142: 145-8.
[http://dx.doi.org/10.1016/j.actatropica.2014.11.011] [PMID: 25438258]

[8]     Souza WD, Martins-Duarte ED, Lemgruber L, Attias M, Vommaro RC. Structural organization of the tachyzoite of *Toxoplasma gondii.* Sci Med 2010; 20(1): 131-43.

[9]     Dubey JP, Kotula AW, Sharar A, Andrews CD, Lindsay DS. Effect of high temperature on infectivity of *Toxoplasma gondii* tissue cysts in pork. J Parasitol 1990; 76(2): 201-4.
[http://dx.doi.org/10.2307/3283016] [PMID: 2319420]

[10]    Dumètre A, Dardé ML. How to detect *Toxoplasma gondii* oocysts in environmental samples? FEMS Microbiol Rev 2003; 27(5): 651-61.
[http://dx.doi.org/10.1016/S0168-6445(03)00071-8] [PMID: 14638417]

[11]    Jones JL, Dubey JP. Waterborne toxoplasmosis--recent developments. Exp Parasitol 2010; 124(1): 10-25.
[http://dx.doi.org/10.1016/j.exppara.2009.03.013] [PMID: 19324041]

[12]    Sibley LD, Boothroyd JC. Virulent strains of *Toxoplasma gondii* comprise a single clonal lineage. Nature 1992; 359(6390): 82-5.
[http://dx.doi.org/10.1038/359082a0] [PMID: 1355855]

[13]    Morgan UM. Detection and characterisation of parasites causing emerging zoonoses. Int J Parasitol 2000; 30(12-13): 1407-21.
[http://dx.doi.org/10.1016/S0020-7519(00)00129-6] [PMID: 11113265]

[14]    de Moura L, Bahia-Oliveira LM, Wada MY, *et al.* Waterborne toxoplasmosis, Brazil, from field to gene. Emerg Infect Dis 2006; 12(2): 326-9.
[http://dx.doi.org/10.3201/eid1202.041115] [PMID: 16494765]

[15]    Montoya JG, Liesenfeld O. Toxoplasmosis. Lancet 2004; 363(9425): 1965-76.
[http://dx.doi.org/10.1016/S0140-6736(04)16412-X] [PMID: 15194258]

[16]    Zhou P, Chen Z, Li H, Zheng H, Lin RQ, Zhu XQ. *Toxoplasma gondii* infection in humans in China Parasites and Vectors [Internet]. 2011;4(165) [cited 2016 Feb 25]. Available from: https://parasitesandvectors.biomedcentral.com/articles/10.1186/1756-3305-4-165

[17]    Amendoeira MR, Camillo-Coura LF. Uma breve revisão sobre toxoplasmose na gestação. Sci Med 2010; 20(1): 113-9.

[18]    Dubey JP. Toxoplasmosis in sheep--the last 20 years. Vet Parasitol 2009; 163(1-2): 1-14.
[http://dx.doi.org/10.1016/j.vetpar.2009.02.026] [PMID: 19395175]

[19]    Innes EA, Bartley PM, Buxton D, Katzer F. Ovine toxoplasmosis. Parasitology 2009; 136(14): 1887-94.
[http://dx.doi.org/10.1017/S0031182009991636] [PMID: 19995468]

[20]    Liu Q, Wang ZD, Huang SY, Zhu XQ. Diagnosis of toxoplasmosis and typing of *Toxoplasma gondii.* Parasit Vectors 2015; 8(8): 292.
[http://dx.doi.org/10.1186/s13071-015-0902-6] [PMID: 26017718]

[21]    Ragozo AM, Yai RL, Oliveira LN, Dias RA, Dubey JP, Gennari SM. Seroprevalence and isolation of *Toxoplasma gondii* from sheep from São Paulo state, Brazil. J Parasitol 2008; 94(6): 1259-63.
[http://dx.doi.org/10.1645/GE-1641.1] [PMID: 18576886]

[22]    Dubey JP, Lago EG, Gennari SM, Su C, Jones JL. Toxoplasmosis in humans and animals in Brazil: high prevalence, high burden of disease, and epidemiology. Parasitology 2012; 139(11): 1375-424.
[http://dx.doi.org/10.1017/S0031182012000765] [PMID: 22776427]

[23]    Guo M, Dubey JP, Hill D, *et al.* Prevalence and risk factors for *Toxoplasma gondii* infection in meat

animals and meat products destined for human consumption. J Food Prot 2015; 78(2): 457-76.
[http://dx.doi.org/10.4315/0362-028X.JFP-14-328] [PMID: 25710166]

[24] Monteiro RM, Pena HF, Gennari SM, de Souza SO, Richtzenhain LJ, Soares RM. Differential diagnosis of oocysts of Hammondia-like organisms of dogs and cats by PCR-RFLP analysis of 70-kilodalton heat shock protein (HSP70) gene. Parasitol Res 2008; 103(1): 235-8.
[http://dx.doi.org/10.1007/s00436-008-0957-9] [PMID: 18398626]

[25] Pena HF, Gennari SM, Dubey JP, Su C. Population structure and mouse-virulence of *Toxoplasma gondii* in Brazil. Int J Parasitol 2008; 38(5): 561-9.
[http://dx.doi.org/10.1016/j.ijpara.2007.09.004] [PMID: 17963770]

[26] Su C, Shwab EK, Zhou P, Zhu XQ, Dubey JP. Moving towards an integrated approach to molecular detection and identification of *Toxoplasma gondii*. Parasitology 2010; 137(1): 1-11.
[http://dx.doi.org/10.1017/S0031182009991065] [PMID: 19765337]

[27] Dubey JP, Gennari SM, Labruna MB, *et al.* Characterization of *Toxoplasma gondii* isolates in free-range chickens from Amazon, Brazil. J Parasitol 2006; 92(1): 36-40.
[http://dx.doi.org/10.1645/GE-655R.1] [PMID: 16629312]

[28] Gennari SM, Esmerini PdeO, Lopes MG, *et al.* Occurrence of antibodies against *Toxoplasma gondii* and its isolation and genotyping in donkeys, mules, and horses in Brazil. Vet Parasitol 2015; 209(1-2): 129-32.
[http://dx.doi.org/10.1016/j.vetpar.2015.01.023] [PMID: 25747488]

[29] de Amorim Garcia CA, Oréfice F, de Oliveira Lyra C, Gomes AB, França M, de Amorim Garcia Filho CA. Socioeconomic conditions as determining factors in the prevalence of systemic and ocular toxoplasmosis in Northeastern Brazil Ophthalmic Epidemiol 2004;11(4):301-17

[30] Santos TR, Costa AJ, Toniollo GH, *et al.* Prevalence of anti-*Toxoplasma gondii* antibodies in dairy cattle, dogs, and humans from the Jauru micro-region, Mato Grosso state, Brazil. Vet Parasitol 2009; 161(3-4): 324-6.
[http://dx.doi.org/10.1016/j.vetpar.2009.01.017] [PMID: 19232473]

[31] McDonald JC, Gyorkos TW, Alberton B, MacLean JD, Richer G, Juranek D. An outbreak of toxoplasmosis in pregnant women in northern Québec. J Infect Dis 1990; 161(4): 769-74.
[http://dx.doi.org/10.1093/infdis/161.4.769] [PMID: 1969458]

[32] Bonametti AM, Passos JdoN, da Silva EM, Bortoliero AL. Surto de toxoplasmose aguda transmitida através da ingestão de carne crua de gado ovino. Rev Soc Bras Med Trop 1997; 30(1): 21-5.
[http://dx.doi.org/10.1590/S0037-86821997000100005] [PMID: 9026828]

[33] Demar M, Ajzenberg D, Maubon D, *et al.* Fatal outbreak of human toxoplasmosis along the Maroni River: epidemiological, clinical, and parasitological aspects. Clin Infect Dis 2007; 45(7): e88-95.
[http://dx.doi.org/10.1086/521246] [PMID: 17806043]

[34] Grigg ME, Sundar N. Sexual recombination punctuated by outbreaks and clonal expansions predicts *Toxoplasma gondii* population genetics. Int J Parasitol 2009; 39(8): 925-33.
[http://dx.doi.org/10.1016/j.ijpara.2009.02.005] [PMID: 19217909]

[35] Dias RA, Freire RL. Surtos de toxoplasmose em seres humanos e animais. Semina 2005; 26(2): 239-48.

[36] Robson JM, Wood RN, Sullivan JJ, Nicolaides NJ, Lewis BR. A probable foodborne outbreak of toxoplasmosis. Commun Dis Intell 1995; 19: 517-22.

[37] Choi WY, Nam HW, Kwak NH, *et al.* Foodborne outbreaks of human toxoplasmosis. J Infect Dis 1997; 175(5): 1280-2.
[http://dx.doi.org/10.1086/593702] [PMID: 9129105]

[38] Bowie WR, King AS, Werker DH, *et al.* Outbreak of toxoplasmosis associated with municipal drinking water. Lancet 1997; 350(9072): 173-7.
[http://dx.doi.org/10.1016/S0140-6736(96)11105-3] [PMID: 9250185]

[39]    Carmo EL, Póvoa MM, Monteiro NS, *et al.* Surto de toxoplasmose humana no Distrito de Monte Dourado, Município de Almeirim, Pará, Brasil. Rev Pan-Amaz Saude 2010; 1(1): 61-6.
[http://dx.doi.org/10.5123/S2176-62232010000100009]

[40]    Sacks JJ, Roberto RR, Brooks NF. Toxoplasmosis infection associated with raw goat's milk. JAMA 1982; 248(14): 1728-32.
[http://dx.doi.org/10.1001/jama.1982.03330140038029] [PMID: 7120593]

[41]    Dubey JP, Graham DH, Blackston CR, *et al.* Biological and genetic characterisation of *Toxoplasma gondii* isolates from chickens (Gallus domesticus) from São Paulo, Brazil: unexpected findings. Int J Parasitol 2002; 32(1): 99-105.
[http://dx.doi.org/10.1016/S0020-7519(01)00364-2] [PMID: 11796127]

[42]    Yai LE, Ragozo AM, Soares RM, Pena HF, Su C, Gennari SM. Genetic diversity among capybara (*Hydrochaeris hydrochaeris*) isolates of *Toxoplasma gondii* from Brazil. Vet Parasitol 2009; 162(3-4): 332-7.
[http://dx.doi.org/10.1016/j.vetpar.2009.03.007] [PMID: 19375864]

[43]    Cabral AD, Gama AR, Sodré MM, *et al.* First isolation and genotyping of *Toxoplasma gondii* from bats (Mammalia: Chiroptera). Vet Parasitol 2013; 193(1-3): 100-4.
[http://dx.doi.org/10.1016/j.vetpar.2012.11.015] [PMID: 23200751]

[44]    de Macedo MF, de Macedo CA, Ewald MP, *et al.* Isolation and genotyping of *Toxoplasma gondii* from pregnant dairy cows (Bos taurus) slaughtered. Rev Bras Parasitol Vet 2012; 21(1): 74-7.
[http://dx.doi.org/10.1590/S1984-29612012000100016] [PMID: 22534951]

[45]    da Silva RC, Langoni H, Su C, da Silva AV. Genotypic characterization of *Toxoplasma gondii* in sheep from Brazilian slaughterhouses: new atypical genotypes and the clonal type II strain identified. Vet Parasitol 2011; 175(1-2): 173-7.
[http://dx.doi.org/10.1016/j.vetpar.2010.09.021] [PMID: 20970257]

[46]    Opsteegh M, Teunis P, Züchner L, Koets A, Langelaar M, van der Giessen J. Low predictive value of seroprevalence of *Toxoplasma gondii* in cattle for detection of parasite DNA. Int J Parasitol 2011; 41(3-4): 343-54.
[http://dx.doi.org/10.1016/j.ijpara.2010.10.006] [PMID: 21145321]

[47]    Opsteegh M, Schares G, Blaga R. Blaga R and van der Giessen J on behalf of the consortium, 2016. Experimental studies of *Toxoplasma gondii* in the main livestock species (GP/EFSA/BIOHAZ/2013/01) Final report. EFSA supporting publication 2016:EN-995, 161 pp.

[48]    de Oliveira LN, Costa Junior LM, de Melo CF, *et al. Toxoplasma gondii* isolates from free-range chickens from the northeast region of Brazil. J Parasitol 2009; 95(1): 235-7.
[http://dx.doi.org/10.1645/GE-1730.1] [PMID: 18578589]

[49]    Dubey JP, Levy MZ, Sreekumar C, *et al.* Tissue distribution and molecular characterization of chicken isolates of *Toxoplasma gondii* from Peru. J Parasitol 2004; 90(5): 1015-8.
[http://dx.doi.org/10.1645/GE-329R] [PMID: 15562600]

[50]    Cristina N, Oury B, Ambroise-Thomas P, Santoro F. Restriction-fragment-length polymorphisms among *Toxoplasma gondii* strains. Parasitol Res 1991; 77(3): 266-8.
[http://dx.doi.org/10.1007/BF00930870] [PMID: 1675467]

[51]    Howe DK, Sibley LD. *Toxoplasma gondii* comprises three clonal lineages: correlation of parasite genotype with human disease. J Infect Dis 1995; 172(6): 1561-6.
[http://dx.doi.org/10.1093/infdis/172.6.1561] [PMID: 7594717]

[52]    Ajzenberg D, Bañuls AL, Tibayrenc M, Dardé ML. Microsatellite analysis of *Toxoplasma gondii* shows considerable polymorphism structured into two main clonal groups. Int J Parasitol 2002; 32(1): 27-38.
[http://dx.doi.org/10.1016/S0020-7519(01)00301-0] [PMID: 11796120]

[53]    Lehmann T, Marcet PL, Graham DH, Dahl ER, Dubey JP. Globalization and the population structure

of *Toxoplasma gondii.* Proc Natl Acad Sci USA 2006; 103(30): 11423-8.
[http://dx.doi.org/10.1073/pnas.0601438103] [PMID: 16849431]

[54]    Ajzenberg D, Collinet F, Mercier A, Vignoles P, Dardé ML. Genotyping of *Toxoplasma gondii* isolates with 15 microsatellite markers in a single multiplex PCR assay. J Clin Microbiol 2010; 48(12): 4641-5.
[http://dx.doi.org/10.1128/JCM.01152-10] [PMID: 20881166]

[55]    Su C, Zhang X, Dubey JP. Genotyping of *Toxoplasma gondii* by multilocus PCR-RFLP markers: a high resolution and simple method for identification of parasites. Int J Parasitol 2006; 36(7): 841-8.
[http://dx.doi.org/10.1016/j.ijpara.2006.03.003] [PMID: 16643922]

[56]    Vitaliano SN, Soares HS, Minervino AH, *et al.* Genetic characterization of *Toxoplasma gondii* from Brazilian wildlife revealed abundant new genotypes. Int J Parasitol Parasites Wildl 2014; 3(3): 276-83.
[http://dx.doi.org/10.1016/j.ijppaw.2014.09.003] [PMID: 25426424]

[57]    Ajzenberg D, Bañuls AL, Su C, *et al.* Genetic diversity, clonality and sexuality in *Toxoplasma gondii.* Int J Parasitol 2004; 34(10): 1185-96.
[http://dx.doi.org/10.1016/j.ijpara.2004.06.007] [PMID: 15380690]

[58]    Lehmann T, Graham DH, Dahl ER, Bahia-Oliveira LM, Gennari SM, Dubey JP. Variation in the structure of *Toxoplasma gondii* and the roles of selfing, drift, and epistatic selection in maintaining linkage disequilibria. Infect Genet Evol 2004; 4(2): 107-14.
[http://dx.doi.org/10.1016/j.meegid.2004.01.007] [PMID: 15157628]

[59]    Mercier A, Ajzenberg D, Devillard S, *et al.* Human impact on genetic diversity of *Toxoplasma gondii*: example of the anthropized environment from French Guiana. Infect Genet Evol 2011; 11(6): 1378-87.
[http://dx.doi.org/10.1016/j.meegid.2011.05.003] [PMID: 21600306]

[60]    Khan A, Dubey JP, Su C, Ajioka JW, Rosenthal BM, Sibley LD. Genetic analyses of atypical *Toxoplasma gondii* strains reveal a fourth clonal lineage in North America. Int J Parasitol 2011; 41(6): 645-55.
[http://dx.doi.org/10.1016/j.ijpara.2011.01.005] [PMID: 21320505]

[61]    Owen MR, Trees AJ. Genotyping of *Toxoplasma gondii* associated with abortion in sheep. J Parasitol 1999; 85(2): 382-4.
[http://dx.doi.org/10.2307/3285654] [PMID: 10219327]

# CHAPTER 2

# Human Congenital Toxoplasmosis

**Italmar T. Navarro[1,\*], Regina Mitsuka–Breganó[1], Selwyn A. Headley[1], Jaqueline D. Capobiango[2], Inacio T. Inoue[2], Antonio M.B. Casella[2], Edna M.V. Reiche[2] and Fabiana M.R. Lopes Mori[3]**

[1] *Centro de Ciências Agrárias, Universidade Estadual de Londrina, Paraná, Brazil*

[2] *Centro de Ciências Saúde, Universidade Estadual de Londrina, Paraná, Brazil*

[3] *Centro de Ciências Saúde, Centro Universitário Filadélfia, Londrina, Paraná, Brazil*

**Abstract:** Notwithstanding, the severity of the sequels and the frequency of occurrence, congenital toxoplasmosis in humans continues to be a neglected disease in several countries, including Brazil. This is partly because a large proportion of infected children are asymptomatic at birth, and consequently are not diagnosed and treated during the first year of life, while most develop ocular and neuro–psycho–motor sequels in early adulthood. The disparity of several management protocols for acute toxoplasmosis has resulted in extreme difficulty for the physicians to make decisions, resulting in many patients being subjected to unnecessary therapies and invasive procedures or are not treated adequately. Another great difficulty lies with the diagnosis, since most pregnant women are asymptomatic when infected, while diagnosis is based on laboratory results, whose interpretation is dependent on several factors, including screening and confirmatory tests and the gestational age when blood sample was taken. Another difficulty is related with the post–natal diagnosis, because in many neonates, it is not possible to detect specific IgM antibodies, and the presence of IgG does not confirm an infection, since these can be passively transferred from the mother to the infant. Faced with this dilemma and based on the work of our group with patients, communities, health services, this team of specialists have accumulated widespread knowledge for the elaboration and implementation of the "Health surveillance program of gestational and congenital toxoplasmosis in Londrina, Paraná, Southern Brazil". This successful program has served as the basis for this chapter.

**Keywords:** Clinical aspects, Epidemiology, Maternal screening, Molecular diagnosis, Neonatal screening, Ocular toxoplasmosis, Prevention, Risk factors, Surveillance program, *Toxoplasma gondii*, Transmission, Treatment.

\* **Corresponding author Italmar T. Navarro:** Centro de Ciências Agrárias, Universidade Estadual de Londrina, Paraná, Brazil; Tel/Fax: +55 43 3371-4485; E-mail: italmar@uel.br

# EPIDEMIOLOGY AND THE IMPACT OF CONGENITAL TOXOPLASMOSIS

Although *T. gondii* occurs worldwide, the prevalence of infection is greater in the tropics than in other regions and is reduced as the latitude increases. It is well established that there are several sources of infection of *T. gondii* and that these vary from region to region, hence it is important to identify the factors that are more associated with infection [1]. The possibility of being exposed to the sources of infection is determined by the socioeconomic and cultural conditions, including the practices of food production, water treatment, hygiene, food habits, exposure to soil, and the climate of the region [2]. Consequently, the knowledge of these factors is important to control strategies efficiently [3].

The prevalence of toxoplasmosis in pregnant women varies in each geographical region: being 0.8% in Korea [4], 10.6% in China [5], 34.1% in Sudan [6], and 75.2% in the Democratic Republic of St. Thomas and Principe [7]. A study conducted in the USA revealed a prevalence of 14.9% among 2,221 pregnant women [8]. In Mexico, the prevalence is considered as low, varying between 6.1 and 8.2% in the city of Durango [9, 10]. In Austria, a prevalence of 36% was identified [11], while the positivity observed in Slovenia was 34% of 21,270 pregnant women [12].

A reduction (from 84% in 1960 to 44% in 2003) in the prevalence of toxoplasmosis in pregnant women was observed in France and this phenomenon was attributed to several factors, such as improved socioeconomic levels, hygienic conditions, better sanitary conditions for animal rearing, feeding of cats with commercial food, and the ingestion of frozen meat. In 2007, 31 laboratories identified at least one case of congenital toxoplasmosis (CT) with the surveillance system from a total of 271 cases. The general prevalence of CT in that year was 3.3 for each 10,000 children born alive [13].

The prevalence of CT in pregnant women in Brazil varied from 31% in Caxias do Sul, Rio Grande do Sul, South, to 91.6% in the State of Mato Grosso do Sul, in the Midwest [14, 15]. Nevertheless, studies that have evaluated the risk associated with the transmission of toxoplasmosis in the different geographical regions of Brazil are scarce [16]. Forty-seven confirmed cases of CT due to the identification of specific IgM anti-*T. gondii* antibodies from 140,000 neonatal blood samples collected on filter paper from several Brazilian cities were described, with an estimated incidence of 1: 3,000 live neonates [17].

A study with 1,250 pregnant women from the State of Rio Grande do Sul, showed that the prevalence of IgG (48.5%) and IgM (0.6%) anti-*T. gondii* antibodies and a rate of transmission of 2.2 in 1,000 live neonates [18]. Another study that evaluated 2,126 pregnant women from the Basic Health System at the Northeastern region of the same State, reported that 74.5% (1,583) were positive to IgG anti-*T. gondii* antibodies, while 3.6% (77) of these samples contained specific IgM anti-*T. gondii* antibodies. Additionally, from the 51 children that were followed up to one-year of age, 50 were asymptomatic, three were congenitally infected according to the serological profile, while one of these had ophthalmic lesions and cerebral calcifications [19].

A study that evaluated 522 seronegative pregnant women for *T. gondii* from Goiâna, Goiás, Midwestern Brazil, described a seroconversion rate of 8.6% (45/522). Seroconversion occurred during the second trimester of pregnancy and the estimated fetal infection was calculated as 34.5: 1,000. These authors revealed that it was the most elevated rate of maternal seroconversion registered in the published literature and highlighted the need for primary and secondary prevention in pregnant women that are at risk [20].

Pregnant women that were attended by the Basic Health Units in Londrina, Paraná, Southern Brazil, demonstrated the seroprevalence of anti-*T. gondii* IgG (49.2%) and IgM (1.2%) antibodies. The age of the pregnant women, per capita salary, educational level, presence of a cat in the residence, and the habit of eating raw vegetables were more frequently associated with the risk of acquiring toxoplasmosis. Alternatively, it was also demonstrated that the ingestion of crude or not fully cooked meat and contact with soil were not associated with the possibility of having toxoplasmosis [21].

In addition, a study that evaluated pregnant women from two cities located at the Western region of the State of Paraná, that were attended by Public Health Service, revealed a prevalence of IgG antibodies of 59.8% in Palotina and 60.6% in Jesuítas [22].

In summary, CT produces an important socioeconomic impact, particularly if the affected infant suffers from mental disability and blindness. In the USA, it is estimated that each year almost 3,000 children are born with CT and that the annual costs associated with the care of these infants varies between 31 - 40 million USD [23].

If the prevalence of the infection is further reduced, the number of seronegative pregnant women is reported higher and therefore there are more pregnant women at a risk of primary infection. However, under this scenario, the level of environmental parasites is also low, resulting in a reduced risk of infection during gestation [24]. In this balance, it is important to investigate the incidence of CT in each population.

# PATHOGENESIS OF CONGENITAL TOXOPLASMOSIS

In CT, the parasite reaches the fetus by the transplacental pathway, resulting in lesions of different degrees that can result in fetal death or severe clinical manifestations. This is directly related to factors, such as the virulence and strain of the parasite, as well as the capacity to produce an immune response and the gestational phase of the infected female [25]. The placenta has a fundamental role in this process, since in addition to act as a natural barrier for the developing fetus, it is a target tissue for the multiplication of *T. gondii* [26]. The placental barrier is more efficient during the early phases of pregnancy and results in the passage of less than 10% of the parasite during this stage, but as pregnancy develops, the placenta becomes more permeable resulting in the passage of 30% of parasites during the second trimester, terminating with 60 - 70% during the final gestational stage, and increases as parturition is reached [25].

Several studies have demonstrated that the risk of a fetal infection increases with the gestational stage, but the associated sequels are reduced as the gestational phase increases, in that the subclinical forms are frequent in infections that occur during the third gestational trimester [27, 28]. Therefore, the severity of infection is inversely proportional to the gestational age, and the rate of transmission is directly proportional to gestational age. Alternatively, ocular lesions are not dependent on the phase of infection, and severe cases of retinochoroiditis can occur even in infections acquired by pregnant women during the second gestational phase.

The rate of transplacental transmission and the risk to develop clinical manifestations can vary in untreated pregnant women and in different geographical regions. Table **1** summarizes the results obtained in a study carried out in France where serologically negative pregnant women were monitored monthly and consequently, the treatment occurred earlier [25].

Table 1. Level of transplacental transmission and the risk to develop clinical manifestations based on the gestational age at which the first infection occurred.

| Gestational age at seroconversion (weeks) | Transplacental transmission* (%) | Risk of the infant to develop clinical manifestations at 3 years of age (%) |
|---|---|---|
| 12 | 6 | 75 |
| 16 | 15 | 55 |
| 20 | 18 | 40 |
| 24 | 30 | 33 |
| 28 | 45 | 21 |
| 32 | 60 | 18 |

*(Table 1) contd.....*

| Gestational age at seroconversion (weeks) | Transplacental transmission* (%) | Risk of the infant to develop clinical manifestations at 3 years of age (%) |
|---|---|---|
| 36 | 70 | 15 |
| 40 | 80 | 12 |

* The diagnosis of the fetal infection was based on amniocentesis done at more than four weeks after maternal seroconversion. Source [30], adapted from [25].

Several authors have considered that the period between the 10th and 26th week as the most critical gestational phase, since at this period the placenta is very large and easily infected and at the same time, the fetus is immature and can suffer important damages [25, 29]. Further, children of mothers that have seroconverted between the 24th and 30th weeks of gestation constitute the group that presents the highest frequency (10%) of clinical manifestations due to congenital infection, since at this gestational stage there is an elevated risk of maternal-fetal transmission and the chances of the appearance of clinical signs are still high [25].

Due to the risk of intra-uterine infection, the clinical scenario of neonatal toxoplasmosis varies from asymptomatic to fatal. The pathogenicity according to the gestational trimester of maternal primary infection, can be classified as follows [31]:

a. Maternal infection during the first trimester: normally results in fetal death.
b. Maternal infection during the second and third trimesters: can result in premature fetus and the Sabin's tetrad: microcephaly, retinochoroiditis, cerebral calcifications, and mental deficiency [32]. The fetus can demonstrate hydrocephalus due to aqueduct stenosis that is frequently associated with obstruction of the drainage of the periventricular system, periventricular necrosis with macro- or microcephaly (in 50% of cases), marked retinal destruction, retinochoroiditis (in 90% of patients with infection), cerebral calcifications (occurring in 69%), and mental deficit or neurological perturbations (60% of all cases) with clinical manifestations of encephalitis and convulsions. The neonate can also have initial lesions, such as disseminated nodules throughout the brain or around necrotic foci; the cerebral ventricles might be dilated and cerebral lesions can calcify. Additionally, ocular lesions can also be observed; these include varying degrees of retinal degeneration and edema, vascular lesions to the choroid, optical neuritis, microphthalmia, nystagmus, strabismus, and iridocyclitis.

Infected neonates can be asymptomatic at birth or exhibit a wide range of nonspecific signs/symptoms, ranging from a systemic infection to the involvement of severe neurological disease and ocular damage as well as auditive deficiency [33]. However, among neonates infected and asymptomatic, more than

85% of these develop retinochoroiditis during infancy or adolescence, and 40% may demonstrate sequels of neurological dysfunction [34].

Consequently, it was suggested that nursing children born from mothers that were confirmed or with a probable infection due to *T. gondii* must be monitored, for at least one year, with clinical evaluation (including ophthalmic and neurological) and periodical serological assays for the diagnosis and treatment of infection as early as possible [35].

In Europe, CT affects 1 to 10 in each 10,000 births; from these, 1-2% have learning difficulties and 2-7% develop retinochoroiditis [36]. In France, 272 cases derived from the National Surveillance Program for Toxoplasmosis were evaluated [13], 11 of these were interrupted during pregnancy due to fetal lesions or fetal death (six abortions and five fetal deaths). In addition, from the number of neonates born alive, 206 were asymptomatic, 28 demonstrated symptoms, and five had serious manifestations of this disease (intracranial calcifications, hydrocephalus and/or retinochoroiditis), with the incidence of toxoplasmosis being 2.9 for each 10,000 infants born alive.

Although a large amount of congenital infections is the result of primary infection acquired during pregnancy, the parasitic transmission can occur in rare cases in immune-competent women that were previously immune and reinfected by *T. gondii* during pregnancy [37 - 40].

A case of CT was described in France that possibly occurred due to maternal reinfection during pregnancy, in which the parasite isolated from the peripheral blood of an infant represented an atypical genotype of elevated virulence that is common to South America but infrequent in France [40]. It is rather likely that reinfection occurred due to the ingestion of horsemeat imported from South America. This hypothesis was tested and confirmed in mice. Consequently, it is recommended that primary preventive measures are maintained even in pregnant women already immunised, particularly those that will be travelling to areas where atypical genotypes of *T. gondii* are known to have occurred [41]. Alternatively, women immuno-compromised and chronically infected with *T. gondii* can transmit the parasite to the fetus due to the reactivation of a chronic infection [42, 43]. Other exceptional cases of vertical transmission by maternal infection that occurred up to eight months before conception have been described [27, 44]. However, in most of these the immune status of the pregnant woman can be explained due to prolonged dissemination of the parasite with consequent infection of the placenta and transmission to the fetus.

## GENOTYPICAL CHARACTERIZATION

Although, there is a single species of the parasite responsible for human and animal toxoplasmosis, the development of molecular tools since 1990 has resulted in the isolation of strains of *T. gondii* in Europe and the USA that can be divided into three genotypes: I, II, and III, being the equivalent of clonal lineages, stable in time and space [45, 46]. However, multilocus and multi-chromosome genotyping of isolates from other continents has revealed a very complex population with great genetic diversity, probably reflecting frequent recombinations between isolates during the sexual life cycle in definitive hosts [47]. This fact has resulted in the formation of recombined isolates (I/II, I/III, or II/III), but also of new clonal haplogroups. Additionally, in some regions, particularly in South America, there are atypical genotypes with several unique polymorphisms that cannot be grouped in any previously defined haplogroup, while isolates type II are considered as being rare [48 - 51].

In Europe, the type II strain is dominant in human and animals [47, 52]. More than 600 genotyped isolates were from the type II genotype [53], including isolates from human CT [46]. The exceptional isolation of atypical strains in France was related to trips made to South America or the ingestion of imported meat [40, 54]. This epidemiological trend is quite similar to that observed in North America, where type II strains are also dominant [55]. However, recent data suggest a greater prevalence of atypical strains in North America than in Europe, and another clonal haplogroup (haplogroup 12) was identified [56].

Until recently it was thought that the immunological status of the patient as well as the pregnancy trimester at the time of maternal infection were the main factors that contributed to the severity of clinical manifestations in adults and the fetus, respectively. However, recent data based on genotyping have changed this concept. Actually, infection is normally asymptomatic and is not questioned when it occurs in immunocompetent individuals from Europe and North America, but the recent experience of French Guiana with the utilization of new genotyping tools, has demonstrated that severe or even lethal toxoplasmosis can occur in immunocompetent patients infected with atypical strains of *T. gondii* [57]. Similar observations were described where cases of retinochoroiditis were considered as being more severe when compared to those described in Europe [58].

The pathogenesis of toxoplasmosis acquired during pregnancy must also be revised. Reinfection with atypical strains can occur in women previously infected, resulting in congenital transmission while the rate of severe congenital infection is greater when women are infected with an atypical or recombined strain relative to type II strains [40].

## DIAGNOSIS OF TOXOPLASMOSIS

The diagnosis of toxoplasmosis is based on laboratory evaluations, since pregnant women do not normally demonstrate clinical symptoms of infection [25]. However, serology is complex and the interpretation of the results is difficult, so there is the need to understand the limitations of each technique and to evaluate the class of immunoglobulins present in association with the gestational phase [59], in an attempt to determine when the infection actually occurred. The risk of vertical transmission in immunocompetent women, with few exceptions, is related to the primary-infection during pregnancy. This primary infection must be confirmed by serological tests, *i.e.*, the change from serologically negative to positive in a patient whose initial screening was negative. While, the appearance of IgG anti-*T. gondii* antibodies permits the confirmation of seroconversion, the isolated finding of IgM can be simply due to the naturally occurring antibodies, an interference or a non-specific reaction.

In practical cases of primary infection, IgM anti-*T. gondii* antibodies appear at the end of the first week, with IgG occurring within less than one month. In the event of the appearance of IgM antibodies during the serological monitoring of a non-exposed patient, it is recommended that the presence of IgM is confirmed with a second evaluation, and with the persistence of IgM antibodies, a weekly control during six weeks is necessary. The occurrence of specific IgG anti-*T. gondii* antibodies during this period then permits the confirmation of seroconversion. In the absence of specific IgG antibodies, it can be concluded that there was interference or a non-specific reaction of IgM antibodies, and in this case, the patient must be considered as being susceptible to *T. gondii*. Specific IgA and IgE anti-*T. gondii* antibodies are also produced during the first week after a primary infection. These antibodies arrive at their highest level within one month and rapidly decrease within a few months after a primary infection.

Normally, the level of specific IgM antibodies is reduced after 1 to 6 months, being negative in 25% of infected individuals within less than seven months [60], but usually remains detectable for one or more years [61]. Alternatively, specific IgA antibodies were initially thought to have a short appearance, but recent studies have demonstrated that this antibody can be detected up to a period of nine months after a primary-infection. Consequently, this antibody cannot be a substitute marker of a recent infection [62].

The periodicity for the detection of specific IgG antibodies depends on the technique utilized; serological methods that use membrane antigens or whole parasites, *e.g.*, the Sabin-Feldman test, indirect immunofluorescence assay (IFA), or the agglutination assay, can identify at an early stage an antibody response that is initially directed against superficial antigens of the parasite. ELISA methods that utilize a mixture of whole and superficial antigens, and which have brand differences, identify IgG antibodies at a later stage. Variations due to the individual immunological response as well as the characteristics of each serological method can affect the kinetics associated with the detection of IgG antibodies, considering that the synthesis of IgG can be detected one to three weeks after the initial increase in the serum levels of IgM. Independent of the method used, the synthesis of IgG antibodies achieves its highest level within two or three months, and thereafter is reduced rapidly and persists throughout the life of the infected individual in residual tissues, which are quite variable between patients [24].

## SEROLOGICAL METHODS AND INTERPRETATION

The Sabin-Feldman dye test, which is based on the lysis of the parasite by specific serum antibodies, in the presence of the complement, was one of the first methods developed and has been used as the gold standard for many years. However, since this technique uses live tachyzoites, it is only used in a few reference laboratories. Other methods that were developed being widely used are the IFA and IHA assays, but these are being substituted by immunoassays with several variations, since these are automated and therefore more adequate for usage in large laboratories. The ELISA capture allows the detection of specific isotopes IgM, IgG or IgE anti-*T. gondii*; this is also achieved with agglutination immuno-adsorption assays (ISAGA), microparticle enzyme immunoassays (MEIA), fluorescence enzyme immunoassay (FEIA), and chemiluminescent with micro-particle assays (CMIA). These different methods are readily available, provided by several services and their results are based on the levels or titer of IgG that cannot be compared between each other, but must be calibrated in comparison with internationally known available serum [63]. Several situations in the routine diagnosis require specialized techniques or procedures for the precise interpretation of the results including:

a. A common problem consists in the correct interpretation of the grey zone of the ELISA-IgG results, *i.e.*, the detection of low levels of IgG. In most cases, these reduced titers in fact corresponds to specific IgG, and must be confirmed by more sensitive assays such as the dye test or Western Blot (WB). A WB assay (WB Toxo GII; LDBio), that is commercially available in Europe but not in the USA, can identify a specific IgG response against several antigens of *T. gondii*, including the major surface protein (SAG 1) of the tachyzoite. This assay has a proven specificity of 100% and 99.2% sensitivity when compared with the dye test [64]. However, these assays are not feasible for use in developing countries due to elevated costs; therefore, it is recommended that paired serology with samples obtained after two or three weeks.

b. Another common difficulty with serological interoperations is related with the detection of IgM antibodies, which must be validated by a gold standard technique ISAGA-IgM [63]. Since most of these methods have elevated specificity, sensitivity is also increased, which is of great concern because most ELISA or ISAGA methods can detect IgM during months or years after an infection. During the monitoring of a cohort of 446 women that contracted toxoplasmosis during pregnancy, it was shown that the detection of IgM antibodies, utilizing ISAGA and IFA, persisted beyond two years was observed in 27% and 9% of all women evaluated, respectively. However, the detection of IgM is not an indicator of recent infection, unless elevated titers are found. Studies performed in reference laboratories in the USA Palo Alto Medical Foundation-*Toxoplasma* Serology Laboratory (PAMF-TSL) have demonstrated that from 451 patients positive for *Toxoplasma* IgM and IgG by other laboratories, 100 (22%) were acutely infected, 335 (74%) had chronic infection, 7 (2%) were not infected, and in 9 (2%) patients the results were not determined. Consequently, the results of *Toxoplasma* IgM and IgG antibodies alone cannot be used to differentiate between acute and chronic infections. Therefore, it is recommended that screened serum be sent to reference laboratories that have the capacity to perform other methods that permit this difference [65]. A method that is frequently used to confirm or not a recent infection is the determination of the IgG avidity [66], which is based on the greater force of the ionic bonds between antigen and antibody in older relative to recent infections [67].

The strength of the force of an antibody bond avidity can be evaluated by an ELISA assay comparing between two patterns of reactions and by using a dissociative buffer (normally urea), which removes the antibody of reduced avidity in a recently acquired infection. The result is then obtained due to the relationship of the level of antibody obtained between the urea treated and untreated reaction; an elevated IgG avidity level permits the exclusion of a recent infection with a precise time-line that is method dependent, but is normally of four months. Since antibody of low avidity can persist for several months in some individuals, the presence does not necessarily indicate a recently acquired infection, but a high avidity is of greater value to exclude infections that have occurred within less than four months [68]. Consequently, the IgG avidity is recommended for women who have realized a first serological evaluation up to 16 weeks of gestation and that are IgM reactive [69]. In routine practice, the IgG avidity test prevents the unnecessary treatment of pregnant women as well as the monitoring and treatment of fetuses and children using invasive methods, which are frequently prolonged until congenital infection can be excluded. In cases of confirmed seroconversion, *i.e.*, the first serology was not positive with further positivity during monitoring; there is no need to evaluate the IgG avidity, since seroconversion confirms an acute infection [70].

The performance of serological tests with two different commercial kits was evaluated: one detected IgA anti-*T. gondii* antibodies and the other evaluated the IgG avidity in a group of pregnant women with acute and chronic toxoplasmosis. These authors demonstrated that the IgA anti-*T. gondii* antibodies had sensitivity of 88.8% with specificity of 85.4%, while the IgG avidity test had sensitivity of 100% with specificity of 92.1%. The authors concluded that the IgG avidity can be used to differentiate between acute and chronic toxoplasmosis using the first serum sample from pregnant women in cases which there is no immunosuppression and the patient is not being treated for toxoplasmosis [71]. Notwithstanding the value of the IgG avidity test, the reactivity to IgM antibodies continues to be the screening assay of choice for cases of acute toxoplasmosis, since this antibody is rarely absent during an acute infection [72].

In Brazil, the extreme difficulty to use the IgG avidity assay as a complementary evaluation is because a large number of pregnant women begins pre-natal health care very late [19, 73], in these cases, the high IgG avidity does not exclude an acute infection at the beginning of pregnancy. Therefore, these pregnant women should be treated and their children monitored until congenital infection is discarded.

An alternative method to determine when an infection occurred lies in analyzing the kinetics of the IgG anti-*T. gondii* titers from two serum samples obtained in a period of two or three weeks in the absence of any specific treatment against toxoplasmosis. Although an increase in the IgG titer is suggestive of an infection acquired within less than two months before the first serum sample, it must be highlighted that therapy can also reduce the IgG avidity or suppress IgG titers [74].

An adequate serological interpretation is the basis to prevent emotional stress of parents with the result of positive IgM antibodies, which actually can indicate an old infection. Due to these difficulties and the need to combine different diagnostic tools, efficient interpretations, and a safe pregnancy, it is recommended by several specialists that positive IgM samples are referred to reference laboratories [24, 65].

Another important factor in the serological diagnosis of toxoplasmosis is the method used to evaluate the antibodies, particularly IgM, in conventional IFA or indirect ELISA, is that there is a competition between IgM and IgG antibodies for the binding antigen sites, which frequently produces false negative results [63]. False positive results can also occur in patients due to the presence of antinuclear antibodies or the rheumatoid factor [75]. Therefore, it is recommended to utilize methods that have IgM-capture antibodies in order to reduce the occurrence of false negative results.

In addition, continuous efforts have been made to develop diagnostic methods to determine the date of infection. These include different approaches, such as the detection of IgM anti-glycosyl-inositol-phospholipid that was associated with a recent toxoplasmosis infection [76], and the utilization of recombinant proteins synthesized from *T. gondii* and evaluated for sensitivity and specificity of IgG using ELISA [77, 78]. Some of these methods have demonstrated an interesting avidity response by allowing the better use of crude antigens to discriminate between acute and chronic infections, but their usage in routine laboratories must be validated by studies evaluating a large number of samples from diverse geographical locations [77, 79].

The diagnosis of toxoplasmosis by serology is complex, has been in continuous evolution, requires a variety of assays, as well as a wide experience to interpret the obtained results. Bessières *et al* (2006) listed several difficulties associated with the interpretation of clinical cases of toxoplasmosis [80] including:

- Positive IgM anti-*T. gondii* up to three years after an acute infection;
- Seroconversion with very low levels of IgM anti-*T. gondii*;
- The presence of nonspecific IgM;
- Delayed IgG anti-*T. gondii* response (two months after detection of IgM);
- Serological reactivation with an increase in the titer of IgG, the appearance of IgA, the absence of IgM, and a strong IgG avidity.

Even with these difficulties, the authors recommended laboratory diagnosis, remembering that diverging results can occur and that these must be defined by the repetition of examinations after a few weeks or the utilization of different methods for the detection of antibodies.

Seronegative pregnant women are susceptible to an infection by *T. gondii*; therefore, periodic serological monitoring until the end of pregnancy is needed to detect maternal seroconversion. This strategy can be used to identify a change in the status of seroreactivity, which provides conclusive information of infection and the period of acquisition, confirming whether the neonate under investigation is at risk of being infected.

Due to the significant number of neonates affected by CT, it has become necessary to understand the clinical and laboratorial characteristics of toxoplasmosis in pregnant women and the time of maternal seroconversion in an attempt to begin an early antiparasitic therapy and to reduce the possibility of alterations in the fetus.

## FETAL DIAGNOSIS

Although several questions have been raised during the last few years relative to the prophylactic therapy of toxoplasmosis to prevent fetal transmission by the usage of spiramycin, it seems as though there are no doubts that the treatment of infected fetuses with an association of pyrimethamine and sulfonamide (or sulfadoxine or sulfadiazine) (PS) can reduce the incidence of sequels in children [81]. However, due to the adverse effects of these drugs, it is believed that this combined therapy should only be administered to pregnant women with a confirmed diagnosis of CT [31].

Conventional evaluations to establish a diagnosis of fetal toxoplasmosis include the direct identification of the parasite by the inoculation of the amniotic fluid (AF) and/or blood from the umbilical cord in mice and/or cell culture. This methodology has specificity of 100% but requires a long period to obtain the result with elevated operational cost and low sensitivity, which has made the utilization unfeasible at routine diagnostic laboratories [82 - 84]. The isolation of the parasite can be done from the peripheral blood (preferentially from the buffy coat) or from centrifuged sediment of the cerebrospinal and AF, bronquialveolar lavage, suspensions of grounded biopsy or placenta specimens.

Recent advances with the knowledge of the genome of *T. gondii* have made it possible to use polymerase chain reaction (PCR) assays to amplify the nucleic acid and consequently detect the parasite even in reduced levels of parasitism [85]. Briefly, PCR can be used to detect *T. gondii* within the amniotic fluid; however, false negative results can occur due to retarded transmission of the parasite to the fetus after the PCR was performed [86]; while false positive results can be associated with the contamination of amplified material from a previous positive assay [87]. Alternatively, in developing countries, such as Brazil, the serological monitoring of pregnant women, when done, is trimestral and can result in a late diagnosis of seroconversion. Consequently, at the time of amniocentesis, parasites might not be detected, a factor that contributes towards the low sensitivity of PCR assays done with this biological material. Differences in the genotypes of strains of *T. gondii* used from each geographical region in PCR assays can also affect the sensitivity of this molecular methodology [88].

In the French program, when maternal infection is acquired during pregnancy, the normal practice is to treat the mother with spiramycin until childbirth or be substituted by sulfadiazine-pyrimethamine only if the toxoplasmosis prenatal diagnosis is positive. The AF is collected after 16 weeks of pregnancy and at least four weeks after maternal infection. The prenatal diagnosis is based mainly on the identification of parasitic DNA, but in most reference centers, the AF is also inoculated in mice. This *in vivo* assay is based on the detection of an antibody response in animals by using the serum collected four to six weeks post-inoculation or by the isolation of the parasite [89], but due to the prolonged period to obtain an immune response and the reduced sensitivity compared to PCR, this technique is reserved mainly for the isolation of strains in epidemiological studies.

Several gene targets have been used in PCR assays, resulting in varying degrees of performance [90 - 92]. The level of sensitivity varied from 65 to 80% with conventional PCR [89, 91, 93], and multicenter studies have identified large differences between each center [94]. The heterogeneity of PCR assays was clearly demonstrated in a European study [95]. Another multicenter study, involving 33 laboratories from 14 European countries and three from outside of Europe, was done to evaluate the performance of the PCR to amplify nuclei acid for the detection of *T. gondii* in a panel consisted of five lyophilized coded AF samples in a range of concentration between 5 to 1000 parasites/ml and a negative control. This study revealed the need to increase the specificity and sensitivity of molecular methods and the acquisition of international reference samples to assist laboratories in the development and validation of their methodologies [96]. The need to standardize molecular methods for the diagnosis of toxoplasmosis was emphasized and the utilization of real-time PCR (qPCR) as a method to standardize all the results was recommended [96]. Additionally, the DNA extraction procedures led to variable efficacy, especially in low concentrations of tachyzoites in AF samples [97].

Among several gene targets, the REP-529, which is repeated 200-300 times within the *T. gondii* genome, has achieved better results [90]. In France, where the prenatal diagnosis of toxoplasmosis is a routine procedure for decades, a special effort has been done to evaluate the performance of diagnostic methods used at reference centers [98, 99]. A prospective multicenter clinical study that evaluated the performance of qPCR with REP-529 has revealed that the parasite was detected in the AF of 47/51 (92%) infected fetuses, thereby confirming the elevated sensitivity of this gene in the prenatal diagnosis of toxoplasmosis [100]. However, this method must be validated for usage in other countries, mainly in South America, where there is a wide variety of genotypes, maternal screening is not compulsory, and there is trimestral serological evaluation (when done) of seronegative pregnant women.

False negative results are probably due to the low levels of parasites in the AF [91, 99]. The sensitivity of prenatal diagnosis is lower when maternal infection occurs during the first gestational trimester compared to those acquired at a later stage, suggesting that vertical transmission could have occurred after amniocentesis [100, 101]. In addition, early maternal therapy can contribute towards the reduction of the parasitic burden detected within the fetal compartment, which can be explained due to the reduced number of parasites quantified in the AF.

It was suggested that qPCR should be used as a prognostic marker, since more elevated concentrations of *T. gondii* in the AF was associated with clinical manifestations in fetus and neonates [91]. However, the results of multicenter studies have demonstrated the failure to reproduce the quantification of the parasite, particularly when the parasitic load is reduced, during the standardization of methods [99].

In countries where the monitoring policy includes prenatal diagnosis, a positive result determines the replacement of therapy with spiramycin to PS. In cases where infection occurs during the third trimester of pregnancy, the therapy with pyrimethamine-sulphonamide should be immediately prescribed and the postnatal diagnosis of CT must be done. Medical induced abortions, in countries where they are permitted, are normally reserved for the cases of severe fetal abnormality identified during ultrasonographic evaluation [24].

Since PCR has limitations of sensitivity, varying from 42 to 97%, and specificity from 87 to 100% based on the methodology used and the sequence of nucleotides used as primers in each laboratory [84, 95, 102 - 104], particularly in countries that do not have reference laboratories, PCR is not recommended for the routine laboratorial diagnosis of fetal infection. It was suggested that this methodology is used in routine diagnostic laboratories only after it has been significantly improved, with the reduction of discording results [96]. Consequently, due to the unfeasibility to provide a fetal diagnosis, therapy with PS must be done after $18^{th}$ week of pregnancy, since CT can produce serious lesions to the fetus [63].

Monthly ultrasonography is recommended for all pregnant women with a suspicious or confirmed diagnosis of acute toxoplasmosis. The ultrasonographic findings are suggestive, but not confirmatory of CT, and include uni or bilateral ventricular dilation, ascites, intracranial calcification and hepatosplenomegaly [15, 63].

## MATERNAL THERAPY

The issue regarding the most adequate maternal therapy is discussed, since no randomized clinical study was done to compare different therapy schemes. The therapy with spiramycin alternating with PS every three or four weeks is adopted in many healthcare programs [105]. However, a retrospective study done in Lyon, France, observed a reduction in the severity of lesions after 1995, which coincided with the substitution of 3-weeks scheme of PS with spiramycin following a positive antenatal diagnosis in favour of continuous PS treatment up until delivery [106].

The drugs used in the therapy of toxoplasmosis are:

a. Spiramycin: indicated during the first gestational trimester in cases of pregnant women with acute infection, due to the incapacity to cross the placental barrier, and therefore, without the risk of inducing iatrogenic fetal damages.
b. Triple scheme: the combination of PS associated with folinic acid is indicated for pregnant women in more than 18 weeks of gestation, since pyrimethamine is potentially teratogenic [30]. The other toxic effect of pyrimethamine is that, by being an antagonist of folic acid, can produce reversible and gradual bone marrow suppression. The suppression of platelets is the more severe consequence, thus pregnant women and children with prolonged use of this drug must be periodically monitored with hematological analyses (red and white peripheral blood cell and platelet counts), and the therapy temporarily suspended if moderate or severe alteration is observed in the hematological evaluation. The concomitant use of folinic acid is indicated to prevent these toxic effects, and the dosage adjusted if necessary. On the other hand, PS treat the infected fetus.

Spiramycin is a macrolide antibiotic that was associated with the reduced frequency of vertical transmission. This drug is indicated for women with acute toxoplasmosis or in suspected cases acquired at the beginning of gestation. However, the efficacy of spiramycin to prevent CT has been placed in doubt by European scientists [107, 108], but these studies are not conclusive and are questioned by others [61]. Until conclusive results with regard to the efficacy of this therapy, many specialists continue to recommend spiramycin for pregnant women with suspected or confirmed acute toxoplasmosis, acquired during the first trimester and the beginning of the second trimester [29, 61, 109]. Nevertheless, this drug must be replaced by the triple scheme after the 18th week of pregnancy [63]. The triple scheme is also indicated for pregnant women diagnosed with suspected or confirmed acute toxoplasmosis during the second or third gestational trimester, especially in cases the fetal infection can not be ruled out.

## PREVENTION AND CONTROL OF CONGENITAL TOXOPLASMOSIS

The serological screening of pregnant women permits the early detection of maternal infection and prenatal therapy with the objective to reduce vertical transmission, or when already occurred, to reduce sequels in the infected fetus. Additionally, screening results in the identification of seronegative pregnant women that are at risk of acquiring a primary-infection and congenital transmission, thereby resulting in the orientation of control measures that can be implemented. However, prenatal screening is not mandatory and differs by country in accordance with the prevalence of toxoplasmosis and health policies.

The elevated prevalence (70%) of toxoplasmosis observed in France in 1970 motivated the implantation of prenatal serological screening during the first trimester of pregnancy in 1985, and was reinforced in 1992 with the implementation of monthly repeated exams in women who were seronegative [24]. In Austria, the prenatal screening program was established in 1975 [110], with bimonthly serology for seronegative women [104], while other European countries, such as Belgium, Norway and a few Italian cities, instituted a program with the serological evaluation of negative pregnant women each trimester. Other countries, such as Poland, Denmark, Sweden, and the USA do not have a prenatal screening system for toxoplasmosis [25]. In the absence of screening, hygiene measures are fundamental to prevent CT and must be widely disseminated between all pregnant women.

In countries where prenatal screening is mandatory, serology must be required as soon as the pregnancy has been diagnosed so that the serological status of the patient can be adequately interpreted and preventive measures must be taken with seronegative women in an attempt to prevent infection. Repeated serology provides the option to initiate a specific therapy as soon as seroconversion is observed and to propose prenatal diagnosis.

Notwithstanding the advantages of prenatal screening, several doubts have been raised relative to the practical aspects:

a. There is no adequate evidence whether the benefits of antenatal therapy to reduce parasite transmission or to reduce fetal damage or newborn sequelae if the transmission has occurred.

b. There are clinical risks associated with the fetal diagnosis when amniocentesis is required. Several studies have identified serious risks associated with fetal loss and other complications such as infections or premature contractions and collateral effects associated with fetal therapy with PS [29, 112], but these effects are lower than the rate of fetal transmission. In the Austrian retrospective study, 1,386 amniocenteses were done between 1992 to 2008 and no conventional complications associated with amniocentesis were recorded [111].

c. The cost and difficulties in the implantation of screening programs, with more elevated costs in countries where the prevalence of toxoplasmosis is lower due to the large number of seronegative pregnant women who must have repeated serological evaluations during pregnancy.

Therefore, the decision to implement prenatal screening in a country must be carefully considered and based on prevalence data, disease load, technical resources, and the cost of diagnosis.

In France, a mandatory prenatal screening includes an initial serological evaluation before the end of the first trimester of pregnancy, and in case of negative results, all pregnant women are being retested monthly, and a final serology is done 2 or 3 weeks after delivery, resulting in approximately seven serological evaluations for each negative woman. This program permits the early diagnosis of seroconversion and adequate treatment to prevent vertical transmission [25]. Spiramycin has been used in France since the 1960s for the primary prevention of CT in the first trimester [113], after that, if prenatal diagnosis with PCR is positive, spiramycin is substituted for the triple scheme and it is considered very efficient to reduce sequels.

During the last decade, contradictory results relative to the efficacy of the maternal therapy to prevent vertical transmission elaborated by several epidemiological studies or retrospective cohort meta-analyses have initiated the debate concerning the importance of screening. A systematic review that included 2,591 studies of CT did not identify any effect suggesting that therapy might reduce vertical transmission [114]. However, some important parameters were absent from these studies, such as the absence of prolonged monitoring (> than 6 months of study) of neonates to discard congenital infection with an elevated degree of confidence; the delay between maternal infection and the onset of therapy; and the absence of an adequate control group. The absence of these factors reduced the confidence of the general conclusions relative to the efficiency of therapy. Similar conclusions were obtained by the European Multicentre Study on Congenital Toxoplasmosis (EMSCOT) that included 1,208 pairs of mother-infant from 11 centres, and did not identify any evidence that therapy reduces the transmission of the parasite but also could not exclude a clinically important effect [107]. The authors recognized several sources of potential biases in the interpretation of the results from this cohort study, such as the differences in therapy protocols, reduced number of non-treated controls (only 106 patients), and the prolonged delay to begin the therapy in countries where serological screening is done in periods of three months. Another meta-analysis study, The Systematic Review in Congenital Toxoplasmosis (SYROCOT) study group, found weak evidence of an association between early treatment started within 3 weeks, and reduced mother-to-child transmission compared with treatments that initiated after 8 or more weeks. This study enrolled 26 cohorts and 1,745 infected mothers (including 307 untreated) [108].

Other than a reduction in vertical transmission, the objective of prenatal therapy is to reduce fetal damage and sequelae in the neonate, when transmission has already occurred. The therapy efficiency can be evaluated by cohorts of patients that have benefited from prenatal screening compared with a non-treated control group. However, as previously discussed, this evaluation will suffer from the absence of adequate non-treated control groups and the necessity of precise recording of the date of maternal infection, since the severity of the fetal infection, and proportionally, the capacity of therapy to reduce sequelae, will depend on when seroconversion occurred. Several studies reveal conflicting results; while the SYROCOT study did not identify any evidence that prenatal therapy reduced the risk of clinical manifestations [108], two prospective multicentre cohorts done in European centres demonstrated that prenatal therapy (spiramycin or PS) was associated with the reduction of intracranial lesions, severe neurological sequels or death [115, 116]. These results are in accordance with the observation that the systematic screening and treatment of pregnant women reduced the level of severe congenital infections in France, where the level of asymptomatic infected neonates is approximately 85% of all births [13].

Alternatively, a study done in Brazil demonstrated that 79.8% (142/190) of children born with CT had ocular lesions affecting at least one eye. During that study, only 5.8% of women were treated during pregnancy [117]. However, the large occurrence of symptomatic cases described in Brazil must be evaluated with caution, since it is known that the *T. gondii* genotypes in South America are more virulent [58].

A recent French study regarding to the efficiency of the prenatal management on the impact of the disease verified that the transmission rate was greater during 1987 to 1991, *i.e.*, before the use of mandatory monthly serological screening, compared to 1992 to 2008 [106].

In order to obtain definite conclusions relative to the efficiency of therapy in the reduction of fetal transmission and sequels, a large number of clinical randomized and controlled trials are necessary. Nevertheless, the development of these studies is prohibited due to ethical considerations, and trails including a non-treated group cannot be done in countries where there are routine monitoring and prevention.

## PREVENTION OF TOXOPLASMOSIS DURING PREGNANCY

Although it is poorly valued, the effective prevention of CT is the prevention of primary infection during pregnancy [36], which can be achieved through good hygienic-dietary practices.

Prevention must be based on the implementation of measures that reduce most of the risks associated with the transmission of toxoplasmosis and must take into consideration the three forms of transmission: 1) tachyzoites that can be transmitted congenitally across the placental barrier, by transfusions, organ transplants, and accidents in laboratories; 2) *T. gondii* cysts by the ingestion of raw or inadequately cooked meat; and 3) oocysts from the soil, plants, and sand boxes, that can be easily disseminated in the environment by transport hosts, such as flies, roaches, worms, and the fur of cats.

The transmission due to the ingestion of cysts depends on the frequency of the ingestion of raw or inadequately cooked meat [27]. Inadequately cooked meat was the main risk factor associated with infection in pregnant women in a case controlled multicentre European study [36]. It was highlighted that the elimination of cysts in meat can be done by thorough cooking at a temperature of 66°C [31]. However, freezing induces a marked reduction in the *via*bility of *T. gondii* in meat, but the total destruction of the parasite depends on the temperature, freezing time, and the type and thickness of the meat. For those persons who do not wish to consume particularly mutton, it is indicated the purchase of frozen meat (at least at -18°C).

Domestic cats are the principal hosts to maintain the biological cycle of *T. gondii*, by being the only host that has all phases of the life cycle of this parasite. Cats become infected due to the ingestion of tissue cysts from infected animals or oocysts from the environment. The infection of cats *via* the ingestion of cysts is very important, mainly in stray or domesticated cats that normally hunt for food. Since these animals defecate in the soil without being noticed, contamination is very difficult to be controlled [31].

However, cats eliminate oocysts once during their lifetime and excretion is restricted to a few weeks. In addition, infective oocysts are not easily fixed to the fur of the cat, since these are removed by the cat before they have attained an infectious potential [118]. Consequently, having a cat at home does not necessarily serve as a risk to acquire toxoplasmosis if preventive measures are taken, such as restriction of feeding cats with raw or inadequately cooked meat, daily removal of feces, and prevent them from hunting [36, 119].

Sand and soil contaminated by the excrement of cats are important and prolonged sources of contamination, and hence not easily eradicated. Flies and roaches must also be controlled since they have been experimentally demonstrated as vectors of oocysts [31]. Although the risk associated with water consumption is not fully elucidated, reports of toxoplasmosis associated with water, mainly non-treated or unfiltered, in countries where surface water is the main source of potable water and where the systems of water filtering are not adequate, are increasingly frequent [120].

Several outbreaks of toxoplasmosis with hydric association were described in developing countries, such as Brazil and India [120 - 122], as well as in developed nations, including North America and Poland [123, 124], suggesting that preventive measures must be reinforced to this specific risk factor and recommended the drinking of bottled water by pregnant women. Additionally, the possibility for the ingestion of water at contaminated lakes and rivers during recreational activities exists, which might explain the large proportion of cases of toxoplasmosis of undetermined origin in pregnant women, as was demonstrated in a study done in Northern USA where this habit is very common [123].

The introduction of new preventive measures associated with the risk from more recently recognized sources of infection, such as unpasteurized or raw goat milk, crude oysters and seafood was also proposed [122].

1. Orientations relative to new preventive measures must be directed towards seronegative pregnant women in countries where there is routine serological screening. Considering the recent information relative to virulent strains of *T. gondii* in some continents, it is recommended that these hygienic measures be adopted by seronegative pregnant women travelling to South America or Africa. Pregnant women should be oriented about hand washing after contact with crude meat, after using soil or sand, and after close contact with cats. In addition, fruits and vegetables must be washed (particularly those that grow in close contact with the soil) before eaten crudely; it must be highlighted that oocysts are resistant to chloride, and as such, the removal of oocysts must be done by mechanical rubbing under running water. Further, pregnant women should not consume raw or inadequately cooked meat, and if she possesses a cat, the sand box must be changed daily, preferentially by another person, and in the unfeasibility of another individual effecting the changes, the pregnant women should use a face mask and gloves. Everyone must be encouraged to maintain cats confined indoors and feed them only with canned food or commercially prepared animal foods. A resume of preventive measures is given at Box 1.

The propagation of these measures depends on public health policy in a given country. Physicians should be at the frontline to provide detailed explanations of the preventive measures to pregnant women or women who are contemplating pregnancy. Oral counselling should be accompanied with written documentations so that the information can be better appreciated, resulting in the changing of risk habits associated with toxoplasmosis.

Evidence suggests that educational health policies can assist in the reduction of the risks associated with CT, but investigations that evaluated educational policies are scarce worldwide [125].

With relation to pregnant women, it is important that serological tests to identify anti-*T. gondii* antibodies be done at the first prenatal evaluation, and in case the pregnant woman does not demonstrate antibodies, she must receive orientation about preventive measures.

**Box 1 - Recommendations for pregnant women to prevent infection by *Toxoplasma gondii*.**

| |
|---|
| • Ingest well-cooked (67° C for 10 minutes) meat |
| • Do not experiment the ingestion of raw or uncooked meat |
| • Freeze all products derived from sheep (-18°C for 7 days) |
| • Stuffed fresh products must be well cooked before consumption |
| • Wash with soap and water all utensils (knives, boards, *etc.*) used during the preparation of meat |
| • Fruits and vegetables must be thoroughly washed and scrubbed under running water |
| • Protect all food from flies and cockroaches |
| • Drink only treated or boiled water |
| • Boil and/or pasteurize goat milk before consumption |
| • Wash hands thoroughly after playing with sand or soil |
| • For those with cats:<br>− Do not feed raw meat<br>− Ask another person to remove the excrement **daily**<br>− Prevent the animal from hunting |

A study done in Belgium demonstrated that health education was associated with the reduction of 63% of maternal seroconversion [126]. While a control study observed that knowledge relative to the risk factors associated with infection by *T. gondii* was almost doubled within four years of educational health [127].

Another factor that must be considered is the efficiency of the diverse vehicles of communication, such as the written press, female magazines, and mass communication. Several authors have identified that orientation done personally by health professionals is more efficient and that printed orientation is insufficient to induce behavioural changes in the risk factors associated with toxoplasmosis [59, 127, 128]; these facts demonstrated the importance of training health professionals so that they can effectively and correctly guide pregnant women on the types of prevention.

In the USA, the knowledge of obstetricians and general clinicians relative to the factors associated with the transmission of toxoplasmosis was evaluated and the results showed that obstetricians have more knowledge about the important factors, such as ingestion of improperly cooked meat and gardening without gloves; however, both groups of professionals inappropriately advised that there must not be any contact with cats to prevent toxoplasmosis [129]. These authors concluded that education based on the risk factors associated with the transmission of toxoplasmosis is necessary for these professionals so that they can adequately orient the population and consequently reduce the level of CT.

The programs of primary prevention must be based on the epidemiological and cultural characteristics of each geographical region. Therefore, it is of fundamental importance for each population, that the principal risk factors, the degree of education, and the strategies to promote health must be based on the knowledge of the risk factors that affect the behaviour of gestating women in each region [8, 59]. Countries that have programs to prevent CT have reduced disease prevalence, confirming the importance of prevention of infection in gestating women [12].

## NEONATAL SCREENING PROGRAMS

The serological screening of neonates was adopted by some countries as a low cost and an alternative method with reduced risks, since screening is still the only form to diagnose subclinical infections in neonates so that late and disabling sequelae can be prevented [130]. In the USA, several specialists [61, 131] have recommended neonatal screening, since the incidence of CT is equal or higher than metabolic and genetic diseases, such as phenylketonuria, congenital hypothyroidism, and congenital adrenal hyperplasia, for which neonatal screening is mandatory in several US states.

Studies have demonstrated that the detection of anti-*T. gondii* antibodies using the filter paper technique identified almost 85% of infected children [70, 130, 132]. While other studies related that only 48.3-55% of the neonates were IgM positive, with variations based on the trimester when seroconversion occurred [133, 134].

## THERAPEUTIC PROTOCOLS FOR MATERNAL TOXOPLASMOSIS

It must be taken into consideration the gestational age and if the patient is under investigation or with a confirmed infection (Box 2 and 3).

**Box 2.** Therapeutic scheme for toxoplasmosis acquired during gestation for patients under investigation for acute toxoplasmosis irrespective of the gestational age [63].

| Patients | Therapy |
|---|---|
| Under investigation | **Spiramycin** (Rovamycin®, tablets 500 mg)<br>Dose: two tablets 8/8 hours, by oral route (fasting). |

**Box 3.** Therapeutic scheme for toxoplasmosis acquired during gestation for with acute toxoplasmosis [63].

| Gestational period | Therapy |
|---|---|
| **First trimester**<br>(1st to 18th week) | **Spiramycin** (Rovamycin®, tablets 500 mg)<br>Dose: two tablets by oral route (fasting), 8/8 hours. |
| **After the 18th week** (until parturition): **triple scheme** | **Pyrimethamine** (Daraprim®, tablets 25 mg)<br>Attack dose: two tablets, 12/12 hours, during two days by oral route.<br>Maintenance dose: two tables, by oral route, one per daily. |
| | **Sulfadiazine** (Sulfadiazine®, tablets 500 mg)<br>Dose: two tables, 6/6 hours, by oral route. |
| | **Folinic Acid** (Leucovorin® or manipulated, tablets 15 mg)<br>Dose: by oral route, one tablet per day. |

In case of immunosuppressed pregnant women, it is necessary to evaluate the titer of IgG anti-*T. gondii*, clinical signs and symptoms, positivity for *T. gondii* using PCR from blood and/or AF samples in order to institute therapy using the triple scheme, if infection is suspected or confirmed, except in the first trimester, when spiramycin is recommended.

## PRECAUTIONS WITH THE TRIPLE SCHEME

Folinic acid is associated with pyrimethamine and must be administered up to one week after the suspension of therapy with pyrimethamine.

Hematological control (peripheral red and white blood cell and platelet counts) must be evaluated during the first week of therapy and thereafter monthly, being treated with sulfadiazine and pyrimethamine to diagnose haematological adverse effects, such as anaemia, thrombocytopenia, leukopenia or pancytopenia. When these alterations are observed, the use of antimicrobials must be suspended for one month and be replaced by spiramycin as well as an increase in the dose of folinic acid.

The activities of aminotransferases (AST and ALT) must be monitored before the beginning and during the first month of therapy. These evaluations must be repeated if there are alterations in the activity of hepatic enzymes, and in case of pregnant women, have pre-existing hepatic disease, jaundice or persistent vomiting. When it is not possible to use PS, the continuous use of spiramycin must be done until childbirth as alternative therapy.

In case of intolerance to any of the previously mentioned therapies, the pregnant woman must be referred to a medical infectologist for alternative therapy.

## POST-NATAL DIAGNOSIS OF THE CONGENITAL INFECTION

All pregnant women with a confirmed or suspected diagnosis of acute toxoplasmosis must have their children examined at the maternity ward so that the investigation of a congenital infection or the beginning of therapy can be initiated. Due to the pleomorphic nature of CT, that can vary from a very frequent subclinical infection to an infection with nonspecific symptoms that are similar to other congenital infections, the diagnosis of CT is more complicated than that of acquired toxoplasmosis [63].

Congenital toxoplasmosis can be confirmed by the serological evaluation of blood samples of the new born babies. However, the serological diagnosis is very difficult because of the high levels of maternal IgG antibodies anti-*T. gondii* that cross the placental barrier and reach the blood of the neonate. The presence of IgM and/or IgA antibodies anti-*T. gondii* indicates a congenital infection, while the absence of IgM or IgA antibodies does not exclude a congenital infection [63]. In these cases, serological monitoring of IgG anti-*T. gondii* must be done until the infant has attained one-year-of age.

## DETECTION OF SPECIFIC ANTI-*T. GONDII* IGM AND/OR IGM ANTIBODIES

The presence of these two antibodies depends on the period during which maternal seroconversion occurred. Specific IgM antibodies are frequently identified in the blood of the newborn when maternal seroconversion occurred during the third gestational trimester, while the detection of IgA antibodies normally occurs due to seroconversion during the first or second gestational trimester [135]. However, confirmatory serological diagnosis of the infection by *T. gondii* due to the detection of IgM antibodies has been identified in 50-75% of all newborns evaluated [63, 70, 136]. In a study performed in Brazil, the seropositivity due to IgM anti-*T. gondii* antibodies in infants with CT was even more reduced, where only 48% of IgM seropositivity was identified [133]. The absence of IgM can be observed when the maternal infection occurs in the beginning of gestation or when the pregnant woman is treated [135]. Therefore, serological monitoring is often necessary to define CT, which delays the diagnosis and causes insecurity to the affected families [137].

The IgG anti-*T. gondii* antibodies present in the serum of the newborn can be produced by the infant or acquired from the mother *via* placenta. The serum levels of maternal IgG antibodies passively acquired are gradually reduced and disappear between six weeks and 12 months, while the serum levels of endogenous IgG anti-*T. gondii*, produced by the infected infant, persist or increase after birth. However, reduction in the levels of IgG normally occurs during the first months of life, even in a latent infection (due to the reduction of maternal antibody before the active production by infants under empiric therapy). Therefore, the exclusion of congenital infection in an infant that is not under therapy can only be confirmed when there are no circulating IgG antibodies. The reduction in the levels of specific IgG antibodies can be used as an exclusion criterion for infection [25]. However, monitoring must not be interrupted before the confirmation of the absence of IgG antibodies. The increase of IgG antibodies in an infant can occur when therapy is suspended (post-therapy rebound effect).

Since there are several difficulties in the interpretation of the results obtained with conventional serological assays for the diagnosis of CT, all laboratory evaluations must be done by repeating the assays with another sample collected a few weeks later or using other assays to identify different classes of antibodies, which can take several months to define the diagnosis. Therefore, different serological methods are still necessary to identify cases of false negative IgM anti-*T. gondii* antibodies.

In the infected fetus, the IgG and IgM antibodies produced against the antigenic determinants of *T. gondii* can be different from those IgG and IgM antibodies identified in the maternal serum. Cases of CT have been diagnosed during the first days of life, using WB when conventional assays for IgM detection have a non-reactive result [63, 138 - 142].

## WESTERN BLOT

In this context, WB can be used to compare the patterns of recognition by anti-*T. gondii* antibodies from the serum of women and their children which will allow to determine if the antibodies are passively transmitted or produced by the fetus or the infant in cases of CT. In a cohort study of 97 infants (14 infected), the seropositivity of IgG antibodies of women and neonates was evaluated using WB, and the results showed sensitivity of 82.4%, specificity of 93%, and positive predictive value of 95.7%. When WB was associated with the presence of IgM and/or IgA for toxoplasmosis using ELISA, the sensitivity was increased to 85.7% [138]. A study reported the sensitivity of 73.5% and the specificity of 73.5% to the WB-IgG and the combination of WB-IgG and WB-IgM increased the sensitivity to 86.5% for the CT diagnosis [143]. Another study compared the sensitivity to identify IgM anti-*T. gondii* serum antibodies using conventional methods (ISAGA and ELISA) with WB for the detection of IgG and IgM, and revealed a sensitivity of 52% and 67%, respectively, and a specificity of 99% and 96%, respectively. When these two methods were combined, the sensitivity increased from 78% at birth to 85% at three-month-of age with the detection of 94% of the cases of CT [144]. Another study, in Brazil, demonstrated the association of IgM using ELISA and WB-IgG increased the sensitivity to 76% [142]. It was suggested that the WB method should be used for the diagnosis of CT in neonates, since the IgG of children recognizes a collection of antigens that is more diversified than those recognized by the transferred maternal IgG *via* placenta [145]. This method is already in use in Greece for the diagnosis of CT [146].

## PCR

The PCR is the diagnostic method of choice for infections of the central nervous system (CNS), with elevated sensitivity and specificity [63, 147] and can be associated with the serology to confirm CT. The utilization of real time-PCR (qPCR) is promising, since the results can be obtained in four hours with sensitivity of 92% and specificity of 100% [148]. However, this method is not available in the routine of most clinical laboratories, since it depends on the standardization of the methodology, in addition to other precautionary measures with the sample to prevent false negative and false positive results. In study at Minas Gerais, Brazil, the sensitivity of PCR for CT was only 48% [149]. Therefore, the diagnosis of CT depends on the clinical signs and the association with several laboratory methods, such as conventional serology (IgG, IgM, and IgA), WB and PCR.

## COMPLEMENTARY IMAGING AND LABORATORY EXAMS

Non-specific laboratory evaluations can also contribute to the diagnosis of toxoplasmosis. These include hematological evaluation, such as peripheral red and white blood cell, platelet counts that is possible to diagnose alterations, such as anemia, thrombocytopenia, reticulocytosis, leukopenia, atypical lymphocytes, and eosinophilia. Eosinophilia is an important laboratory finding for the differential diagnosis of toxoplasmosis.

Biochemistry analyses include the evaluation of hyperbilirubinemia and the increased activity of hepatic enzymes, such as aminotransferases AST and ALT.

In the cerebrospinal fluid (CSF) it is possible to observe pleocytosis with a predominance of lymphocytes and monocytes. The accumulation of eosinophils and proteins in the CSF are characteristic alterations of toxoplasmosis.

In the ultrasonography of the brain, ventricular dilations and cerebral calcifications can be identified. Computed tomography of the brain, when available, is very useful to observe ventricular dilations and cerebral calcifications.

Ophthalmological fundoscopy is important to visualize signs of uveitis and retinochoroiditis.

## INFANT THERAPY

The therapy of an infant with suspected or confirmed CT, must be done since birth, with the triple scheme: pyrimethamine, sulfadiazine, and folinic acid. The therapy must be stopped in cases where the infection was discarded, while in confirmed cases of CT, therapy must be extended until the infant is one year old [63]. One of the benefits of the treatment of CT is the reduction of neurological and ocular sequels in infected children [150, 151].

A cohort study done in children with CT that were not treated during the first year of life demonstrated that 72% of these developed new chorioretinal lesions, mainly from mid-adolescent [152]. Similar results were described in children with CT, without ocular lesions and that were treated for only one month or at least during the first year of life [34, 153].

Alternatively, in another longitudinal study with children treated during the first year of life, it was verified that only 31% developed new ocular lesions, even though they initially had more severe ocular, neurological and systemic disease [154] than the children from a previous study [152]. Although the cohort of these two studies cannot be compared, the results suggest that therapy during the first year of life significantly reduces the appearance of ocular lesions.

Among the adverse effects of therapy with sulfadiazine and pyrimethamine, neutropenia due to medullar toxicity is worrisome [63]. Research studies have observed moderate and severe neutropenia in few cases, most of these patients were medicated for other coinfections with zidovudine and ganciclovir, and the adverse effects were corrected with the temporary replacement of these drugs with spiramycin and an increase in the dose of folinic acid [133]. In North America, reverse neutropenia was also observed in patients treated with daily doses of pyrimethamine during two or until six months [150].

Considering that the triple scheme is efficient to control the tachyzoites of *T. gondii*, but not adequate for latent cysts, these patients must be monitored for a longer period due to the risk of reactivation of ocular toxoplasmosis and CNS infections [63].

# ROUTINE APPROACH FOR THE DIAGNOSIS OF TOXOPLASMOSIS IN CHILDREN

## Serological Evaluation

Serological assessment must be done in all neonates that are considered with a suspected or confirmed infection by *T. gondii*. Serological evaluation is indispensable, since most cases of CT are asymptomatic.

## Classification of cases based on serology [155]

A - Suspected cases

• Children that are asymptomatic or not, and whose mother had toxoplasmosis during gestation;
• Children born with signs or symptoms of the disease: icterus, lymphadenopathy, microcephaly, hydrocephalus, anemia, convulsions, reduced body weight, prematurity, retinochoroiditis, cerebral calcifications, nystagmus, strabismus, iridocyclitis, alterations to the cerebrospinal fluid, and children with reactive IgG anti-*T. gondii* antibodies.

B - Confirmed cases; children symptomatic or not with at least one of the following situations:

• Reactive IgM or IgA anti-*T. gondii* after one week alive;
• Persistently elevated (or increasing) serum levels of IgG anti-*T. gondii*;
• Children with *T. gondii* confirmed in placental or fetal tissue by histopathology, or by isolation using cell culture or bioassay;
• Children whose mother have positive results PCR for *T. gondii* in AF.

C - Cases under investigation

• Children with declining serum levels of IgG or IgM anti-*T. gondii* non-reactive after the seventh day alive.

D - Discarded cases

• Children that are non-reactive for IgM anti-*T. gondii* and with two non-reactive IgG anti-*T. gondii* results within an interval of at least three weeks and without therapy for more than six months ago.

Recently classified as proven congenital toxoplasmosis [156, 157]:

• Children with reactive IgM and/or IgA anti-*T. gondii* antibodies between two days and six months-of age. The detection of IgA anti-*T. gondii* has the same significance as that of IgM anti-*T. gondii*, even though some studies have indicated a more elevated sensitivity associated with IgA antibodies. However, serological assays to detect IgA anti-*T. gondii* antibodies are not frequently used.

- Children that, during monitoring, maintain the persistence of IgG anti-*T. gondii* antibodies after 12 months-of-age, irrespective of the presence of signs or symptoms of toxoplasmosis.
- Children born from mothers with acquired toxoplasmosis during pregnancy, irrespective of signs or symptoms of toxoplasmosis, with the demonstration of vertical transmission due to paired serological evaluations of the mother with titers in the child that are fourfold or more than that of the maternal titers.
- Children with signs and/or symptoms suggestive of CT, whose mothers have reactive IgG anti-*T. gondii* antibodies, after exclusion of other possible causes, such as syphilis, cytomegalovirus, and rubella.
- Children whose mothers are PCR positive for *T. gondii* in the AF.

### Therapeutic protocol for congenital toxoplasmosis

The therapy for CT is divided into four protocols (Box 4, 5, 6, and 7).

**Box 4.** Therapeutic protocol for asymptomatic children born from mothers with acute infection confirmed or suspected during pregnancy [63].

| Period | Therapy |
|---|---|
| During the first months (until the diagnosis definition) | **Pyrimethamine** (Daraprim®)<br>Attack dose: 2 mg/kg/day, 12/12 hours, during two days; by oral route.<br>Maintenance dose: 1 mg/kg/day (maximum de 25 mg), once per day, by oral route. |
| | **Sulfadiazine** (Sulfadiazine®)<br>Dose: 100 mg/kg/day, 12/12 hours, by oral route. |
| | **Folinic acid** (Leucovorin® or manipulated)<br>Dose: 10 - 15 mg, every three days, by oral route. |

- In case of toxicity, see the therapeutic protocol for children at Box 6.

### Observations

a. These drugs can be manipulated in solution of sugar suspensions at 10%; be careful with formulations and the maximum validity of seven days, under refrigeration at the following concentrations: sulfadiazine, 100 mg/ml; pyrimethamine, 2 mg/ml; folinic acid, 10 mg/ml.

b. The advantage of these suspensions is the ease of administration, but for some children, macerated tablets are more palatable.

c. Due to its residual effect, maintain folinic acid for one week after completing the usage of pyrimethamine.

d. Asymptomatic pre-term neonates: normal physical evaluation and normal laboratory examinations (including CSF), normal USG or CT of the cranium, and a normal ophthalmic examination and case of doubt with the maternal diagnosis (suspected case), begin therapy with spiramycin (dose:100 mg/kg/day; 12/12 hours), until the diagnosis has been confirmed.

**Box 5. Therapeutic protocol children with confirmed congenital toxoplasmosis [63].**

| Period | Therapy |
|---|---|
| Up to two months of age | **Pyrimethamine** (Daraprim®)<br>Attack dose: 2 mg/kg/day, 12/12 hours, during two days; by oral route.<br>Maintenance dose: 1 mg/kg/day (maximum of 25 mg), once per day, by oral route. |
| | **Sulfadiazine** (Sulfadiazine®)<br>Dose: 100 mg/kg/day, 12/12 hours, by oral route. |
| | **Folinic acid** (Leucovorin® 15 mg capsules or manipulated)<br>Dose: 10 - 15 mg every three days, by oral route. |
| The following 10 months to-one-year of age. | **Pyrimethamine** (Daraprim®)<br>Dose: 1 mg/kg/day (maximum of 25 mg).<br>On Mondays, Wednesdays, and Fridays, always a single dose, by oral route. |
| | **Sulfadiazine** (Sulfadiazine® 500 mg)<br>Dose: 100 mg/kg/day, 12/12 hours, by oral route. |
| | **Folinic acid** (Leucovorin® 15 mg or manipulated)<br>Dose: 10 - 15 mg, every three days, by oral route. |

• In serious cases (with neurological symptoms and/or > one ocular and/or > three intracranial calcifications), the daily treatment can be extended with pyrimethamine between four and five months, and later administered in alternative days until the treatment is completed [41].

**Box 6. Therapeutic scheme for children with serious medullar toxicity [63].**

| Patient | Therapy |
|---|---|
| (Hemoglobin > 8g/dL; Neutrophils > 500/mm³; Platelets > 50.000 mm³) | Increase the dose of **Folinic Acid** to 15-30 mg/day. |
| | **Spiramycin** (Rovamycin®)<br>Until laboratory stabilization of results.<br>Dose: 100 mg/kg/day, 12/12 hours, by oral route. |

**Observations**: Considering that spiramycin can cause QT prolongation, an electrocardiograph (ECG) must be done on the first day of using spiramycin, and thereafter, every 15 days until 45 days of age. If it is necessary to maintain the usage of spiramycin for a longer time, a monthly ECG should be performed, if there are no other alterations or clinical complaints.

**Box 7. Therapeutic protocol for children with active retinochoroiditis and/or protein (>1 g/dL) within the cerebrospinal fluid [63].**

| Period | Therapy |
|---|---|
| Add to the triple scheme until regression of the inflammatory ocular process and/or protein within the CSF < 1 g/dl, with gradual reduction of dose until eventual suspension. | **Prednisone** (Meticorten®, 5 mg and 20 mg capsules) **or Prednisolone** (20 mg capsule, suspension with 1 mg/ml or 3 mg/ml). Dose: 1 mg/kg/day, 12/12 hours, by oral route (associated with the triple scheme). |

## EVALUATION OF MEDULLAR TOXICITY

Synergically, PS, inhibits the sequential steps of the biosynthesis of the equivalent of folic acid required by *T. gondii* and their daily utilization implies in adverse hematological effects. Therefore, it is indispensable that this therapy be accompanied by the periodical evaluation of peripheral red and white blood cells and platelet counts. In addition, folinic acid must be administered simultaneously, as preventive measures for these adverse effects, since mammals, unlike *T. gondii*, are able to use acid folinic (see therapeutic protocols).

If the patient shows severe medullar toxicity, such as leukopenia, neutropenia, thrombocytopenia or pancytopenia during hematological monitoring, the therapy with sulfadiazine and pyrimethamine must be interrupted until the parameters of the laboratory evaluations are normalized. During this period, the therapy must be with the utilization of spiramycin (Box 6).

In the event of an intercurrent febrile viral infection, the control of the white blood cell counts must be more frequent, since viral infections have a tendency to induce a reduction in the number of neutrophils (neutropenia). Neutrophils count:

- Higher than $1,000/mm^3$: medication with the triple scheme is maintained.
- Between 500 to $900/mm^3$: folinic acid is increased to 15-30 mg/day, with weekly control of hemogram.
- Lower than $500/mm^3$; PS is suspended, begin with spiramycin and folinic acid is increased to 15-30 mg/day, with weekly control of hemogram. The triple scheme is reintroduced when the neutrophilic count is higher than $1,000/mm^3$.

Observation: Patients with neurological impairment and with neutrophils between 500 to $1,000/mm^3$ were observed sulfadiazine was suspended and clindamycin and pyrimethamine were used, the dose of folinic acid was doubled, and a weekly hematological control was performed.

## Adverse Reactions

- Pyrimethamine: Depression of the bone marrow (gradual effect, reversible, and dose dependent), bleeding dyscrasias, folic acid deficiency, megaloblastic anemia, and rarely exanthema, vomiting, convulsions, eosinophilia and shock.
- Sulfadiazine: Crystalluria, hemolytic anaemia, agranulocytosis, and thrombocytopenia (reversible in most cases), and hypersensitivity reactions, such as exanthema.
- Spiramycin: Gastrointestinal alterations, including diarrhea, vomiting, nauseas, abdominal pain and allergic reactions and QT prolongation.

## APPROACHES

### Maternity

A. Clinical evaluation (Pediatric Infectious Diseases Specialist), ophthalmic and neurological (if neurological alterations are present).
  ◦ Analysis of otoacoustic emissions (done preferentially during the first month of life) in all children.
B. Laboratory evaluation
  ◦ Red and white blood cell counts, platelet counts, total and fractional bilirubin, aminotransferases (AST and ALT) and evaluation of CSF;
  ◦ Ultrasonography or computerized tomography;
  ◦ Serology: detection of IgG and IgM anti-*T. gondii* IgG;
  ◦ Begin empiric therapy until the confirmation of diagnosis.

### Outpatient

A. Return within one week of medication use with results of red and white blood cell counts, platelet counts. Maintenance of the empiric therapy.
B. Return within two weeks:
  ◦ Solicit: red and white blood cell counts, platelet counts, aminotransferases (AST and ALT), anti-*T. gondii* serology (IgG and IgM)
  ◦ Maintenance of empiric therapy
C. Return after 30 days of life:
  ◦ Maintenance of empiric therapy
  ◦ Requirement: red and white blood cell counts, platelet counts within 45 days and thereafter, monthly
  ◦ AST and ALT based on the evolution of the disease are required,
  ◦ CSF analysis as a control if the first sample was altered is required;
  ◦ Anti-*T. gondii* serology (IgG and IgM) for the inconclusive cases is required,

and when necessary, repeated in intervals of three weeks. For confirmed cases, serology with one year of therapy was repeated within 15 months of life;

- Children whose diagnosis is discarded and the therapy interrupted, serology for toxoplasmosis must be done every two months until a negative IgG anti-*T. gondii* is obtained from two serial samples;
- Other congenital or perinatal infections with serologic evaluations for HIV, Cytomegalovirus, Syphilis, Rubella, and Herpes simplex are excluded.
- Children with ventricular dilation at the initial evaluation: refer to a neuropediatric evaluation that will define the periodicity of the ultrasonography and computerized tomography of the cranium;
- Audiometric evaluation with Evoked Potential Analysis, if the neonatal screening was altered or unavailable at the maternity.

D. Returns up to one year of age:
  - Monthly returns until the completion of one year of therapy;
  - Monitoring of cephalic perimeter;
  - Neuropediatric evaluations:
  - Monthly ophthalmic evaluations until the exclusion of congenital infection;
  - Audiometric evaluation with Evoked Potential Analysis.

E. Annual return for clinical evaluation until five-years-of age:
  - Concomitant follow-up with other medical specialities

F. Ophthalmic monitoring in children with confirmed congenital toxoplasmosis:
  - Trimestral evaluation until 18 months of age:
  - Semestral until five years of age;
  - Annual until adolescence.

G. Register on the health card of the child all results of laboratory evaluations, including time of sample collection, methods used in the laboratory evaluation and the respective reference values, the time of treatment started, and the therapeutic protocol used.

  Cases under suspicion, confirmed and in investigation must be notified to the Local Epidemiological Surveillance Unit, where investigation form for toxoplasmosis will be filled.

## OPHTHALMOLOGICAL EXAMINATION OF THE PREGNANT WOMAN AND CHILD DIAGNOSED WITH CONGENITAL TOXOPLASMOSIS OR SUSPECTED SYSTEMIC TOXOPLASMOSIS

Ocular toxoplasmosis is the main cause of uveitis in several countries where the prevalence of toxoplasmosis is elevated. In Brazil, an average of 65.8% of patients are seropositive to *T. gondii*, which contrast the 10.8% of seroprevalence in the USA [2, 158]. The clinical aspects of ocular toxoplasmosis are widespread, with retinochoroiditis being the most frequent manifestation in addition to a characteristic area of retinal necrosis associated with vitritis. There are other less common manifestations, such as neuroretinitis, external punctate retinitis, and even scleritis. In turn, these alterations promote complications, including cataracts, sub-macular neovascularization, retinal detachment, and loss of central vision. Frequently in children with the loss of central vision, there is nystagmus and strabismus, in addition to the more common bilateral involvement and microphthalmia.

All pregnant women with diagnosed or suspected toxoplasmosis must be forwarded to a reference uveitis service for a complete ophthalmic evaluation. The diagnosis of the ocular lesion is achieved by a thorough study that includes visual acuity, assessment of pupillary reflexes, complete biomicroscopy and detailed examination of the retina *via* retinal mapping, and can be extended to the analysis of images with fluorescein angiography, optical coherence tomography, and even ocular ultrasonography [29] (Fig. **1**).

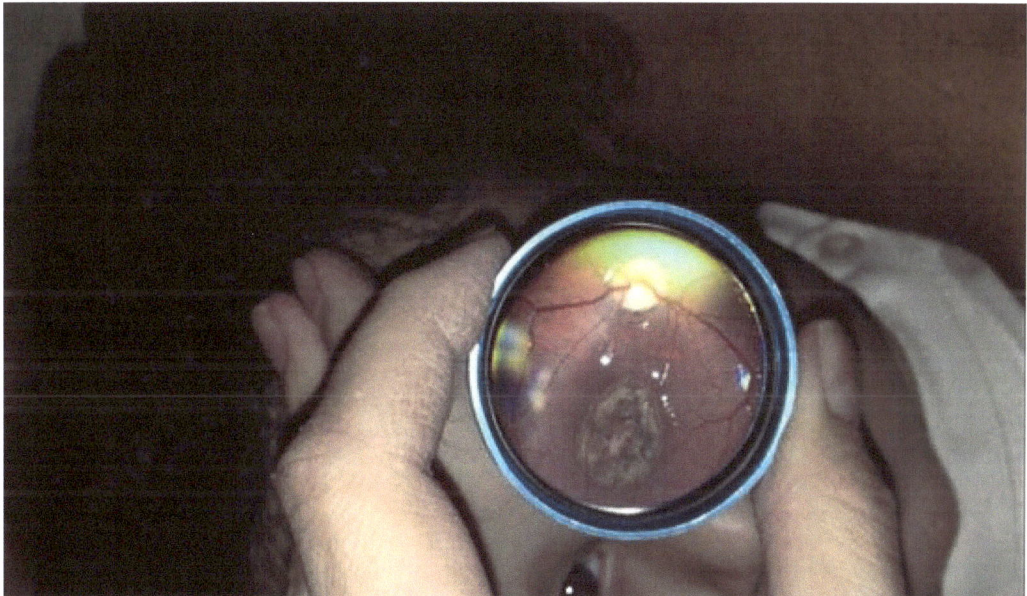

**Fig. (1).** Retinography of an infant with congenital toxoplasmosis done with mobile equipment.

The newborn child of a pregnant woman with a suspected or confirmed diagnosis of toxoplasmosis must be carefully evaluated from an ophthalmic perspective; actually, an ophthalmic screening can produce a diagnosis of ocular toxoplasmosis as outlined in an extensive study carried out in the State of Minas Gerais, Southeastern Brazil. During this study, 146,307 children were screened between November, 2006 and May, 2007, and 178 neonates with CT were identified [159].

While the severity of the clinical manifestations is directly related to the gestational trimester when the fetus was infected from an ocular perspective, the alterations are not totally dependent on the gestational age. In Brazil, the risk of retinochoroiditis, the most common sequelae that persist for several years, occurs in an average of 29 -100% of cases, being bilateral 12-84% of these. Other frequent lesions in these cases include microphthalmia (9-25%), strabismus (12-60%), nystagmus (3-47%), cataract (1-14%) and vitritis (3-50%) [160 - 163].

The clinical ocular alterations observed at the University Hospital, Universidade Estadual de Londrina, Southern Brazil, between January 2000 and January 2010 were primarily retinochoroiditis (55%), in addition to strabismus, vitritis, congenital cataracts, and nystagmus (Fig. **2**). When the occurrence of retinochoroiditis is very common, the macular involvement (Fig. **3**) may restrict the visual acuity of the affected child [133].

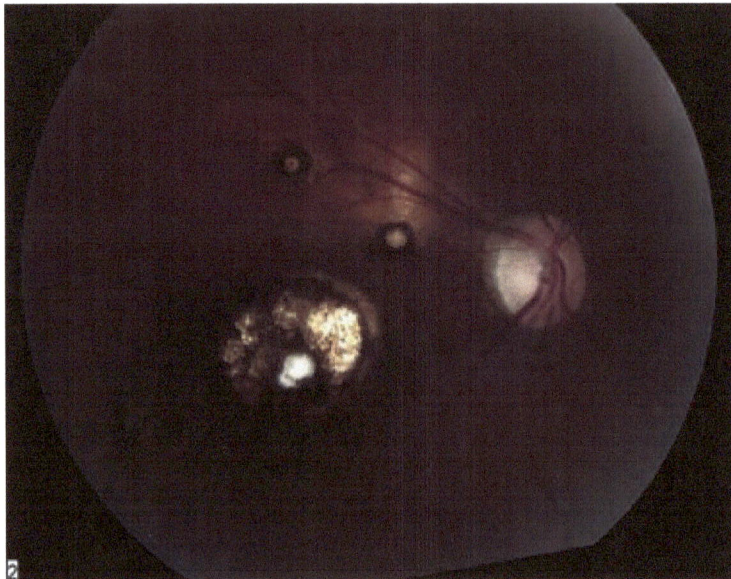

**Fig. (2).** Retinography of an infant with congenital toxoplasmosis demonstrating the ocular recurrence. Source: Dr. Antonio Marcelo Barbante Casella.

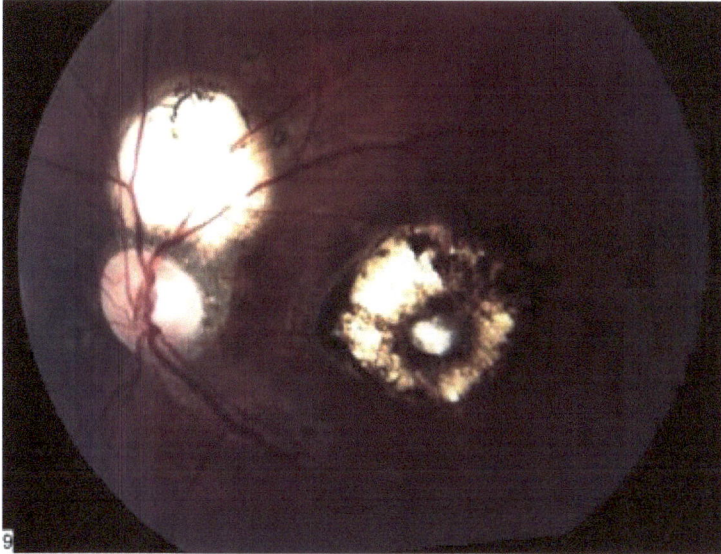

**Fig. (3).** Retinography of an infant with congenital toxoplasmosis demonstrating the macular involvement.
Source: Dr. Antonio Marcelo Barbante Casella.

Once congenital ocular toxoplasmosis is diagnosed in the neonate, prolonged antimicrobial therapy with antibiotics must be performed, since ocular recurrences are more frequent in non-treated cases [152, 154].

## CONSENT FOR PUBLICATION

Not applicable.

## CONFLICT OF INTEREST

The authors declare no conflict of interest, financial or otherwise.

## ACKNOWLEDGEMENTS

Declared none.

## REFERENCES

[1]     Petersen E, Vesco G, Villari S, Buffolano W. What do we know about risk factors for infection in humans with *Toxoplasma gondii* and how can we prevent infections? Zoonoses Public Health 2010; 57(1): 8-17.
[http://dx.doi.org/10.1111/j.1863-2378.2009.01278.x] [PMID: 19744301]

[2]     Jones JL, Kruszon-Moran D, Sanders-Lewis K, Wilson M. *Toxoplasma gondii* infection in the United States, 1999 2004, decline from the prior decade. Am J Trop Med Hyg 2007; 77(3): 405-10.
[PMID: 17827351]

[3]     Edelhofer R, Prossinger H. Infection with *Toxoplasma gondii* during pregnancy: seroepidemiological

studies in Austria. Zoonoses Public Health 2010; 57(1): 18-26.
[http://dx.doi.org/10.1111/j.1863-2378.2009.01279.x] [PMID: 19744300]

[4]     Song KJ, Shin JC, Shin HJ, Nam HW. Seroprevalence of toxoplasmosis in Korean pregnant women. Korean J Parasitol 2005; 43(2): 69-71.
[http://dx.doi.org/10.3347/kjp.2005.43.2.69] [PMID: 15951643]

[5]     Liu Q, Wei F, Gao S, *et al. Toxoplasma gondii* infection in pregnant women in China. Trans R Soc Trop Med Hyg 2009; 103(2): 162-6.
[http://dx.doi.org/10.1016/j.trstmh.2008.07.008] [PMID: 18822439]

[6]     Elnahas A, Gerais AS, Elbashir MI, Eldien ES, Adam I. Toxoplasmosis in pregnant Sudanese women. Saudi Med J 2003; 24(8): 868-70.
[PMID: 12939674]

[7]     Hung CC, Fan CK, Su KE, *et al.* Serological screening and toxoplasmosis exposure factors among pregnant women in the Democratic Republic of Sao Tome and Principe. Trans R Soc Trop Med Hyg 2007; 101(2): 134-9.
[http://dx.doi.org/10.1016/j.trstmh.2006.04.012] [PMID: 17113117]

[8]     Jones JL, Kruszon-Moran D, Wilson M, McQuillan G, Navin T, McAuley JB. *Toxoplasma gondii* infection in the United States: seroprevalence and risk factors. Am J Epidemiol 2001; 154(4): 357-65.
[http://dx.doi.org/10.1093/aje/154.4.357] [PMID: 11495859]

[9]     Alvarado-Esquivel C, Torres-Castorena A, Liesenfeld O, *et al.* Seroepidemiology of *Toxoplasma gondii* infection in pregnant women in rural Durango, Mexico. J Parasitol 2009; 95(2): 271-4.
[http://dx.doi.org/10.1645/GE-1829.1] [PMID: 18922040]

[10]    Alvarado-Esquivel C, Sifuentes-Alvarez A, Narro-Duarte SG, *et al.* Seroepidemiology of *Toxoplasma gondii* infection in pregnant women in a public hospital in northern Mexico. BMC Infect Dis 2006; 6: 113.
[http://dx.doi.org/10.1186/1471-2334-6-113] [PMID: 16839423]

[11]    Aspöck H. Prevention of congenital toxoplasmosis in Austria. Arch Pediatr 2003; 10 (Suppl. 1): 16-7.
[PMID: 12802957]

[12]    Logar J, Petrovec M, Novak-Antolic Z, *et al.* Prevention of congenital toxoplasmosis in Slovenia by serological screening of pregnant women. Scand J Infect Dis 2002; 34(3): 201-4.
[http://dx.doi.org/10.1080/00365540110080386] [PMID: 12030394]

[13]    Villena I, Ancelle T, Delmas C, *et al.* Toxosurv network and National Reference Centre for Toxoplasmosis. Congenital toxoplasmosis in France in 2007: first results from a national surveillance system. Euro Surveill 2010; 15(25): 15. [25 ].
[http://dx.doi.org/10.2807/ese.15.25.19600-en] [PMID: 20587361]

[14]    Detanico L, Basso RM. Toxoplasmose: perfil sorológico de mulheres em idade fértil e gestantes. Rev Bras Anal Clin 2006; 38: 15-8.

[15]    Figueiró-Filho EA, Lopes AHA. Acute toxoplasmosis: study of the frequency, vertical transmission rate and the relationship between maternal-fetal diagnostic tests during pregnancy in a Central-Western state of Brazil. Rev Bras Ginecol Obstet 2005; 27: 442-9.

[16]    Carellos EV, de Andrade GM, Vasconcelos-Santos DV, *et al.* UFMG Congenital Toxoplasmosis Brazilian Group. Adverse socioeconomic conditions and oocyst-related factors are associated with congenital toxoplasmosis in a population-based study in Minas Gerais, Brazil. PLoS One 2014; 9(2): e88588.
[http://dx.doi.org/10.1371/journal.pone.0088588] [PMID: 24523920]

[17]    Neto EC, Anele E, Rubim R, *et al.* High prevalence of congenital toxoplasmosis in Brazil estimated in a 3-year prospective neonatal screening study. Int J Epidemiol 2000; 29(5): 941-7.
[http://dx.doi.org/10.1093/ije/29.5.941] [PMID: 11034982]

[18]    Mozzatto L, Procianoy RS. Incidence of congenital toxoplasmosis in southern Brazil: a prospective

study. Rev Inst Med Trop São Paulo 2003; 45(3): 147-51.
[http://dx.doi.org/10.1590/S0036-46652003000300006] [PMID: 12870064]

[19]  Spalding SM, Amendoeira MR, Ribeiro LC, Silveira C, Garcia AP, Camillo-Coura L. Prospective study of pregnants and babies with risk of congenital toxoplasmosis in municipal district of Rio Grande do Sul. Rev Soc Bras Med Trop 2003; 36(4): 483-91.
[http://dx.doi.org/10.1590/S0037-86822003000400009] [PMID: 12937726]

[20]  Avelino MM, Campos D Jr, do Carmo Barbosa de Parada J, de Castro AM. Medical School of the Federal University of Goiás; Institute of Tropical Pathology and Public Health of the Federal University of Goiás; National Foundation of Support to Research; State Secretary of Health of Goiás; Municipal Secretary of Health of Goiânia. Pregnancy as a risk factor for acute toxoplasmosis seroconversion. Eur J Obstet Gynecol Reprod Biol 2003; 108(1): 19-24.
[http://dx.doi.org/10.1016/S0301-2115(02)00353-6] [PMID: 12694964]

[21]  Lopes FM, Mitsuka-Breganó R, Gonçalves DD, *et al.* Factors associated with seropositivity for anti-*Toxoplasma gondii* antibodies in pregnant women of Londrina, Paraná, Brazil. Mem Inst Oswaldo Cruz 2009; 104(2): 378-82.
[http://dx.doi.org/10.1590/S0074-02762009000200036] [PMID: 19430668]

[22]  Bittencourt LH, Lopes-Mori FM, Mitsuka-Breganó R, *et al.* Seroepidemiology of toxoplasmosis in pregnant women since the implementation of the Surveillance Program of Toxoplasmosis Acquired in Pregnancy and Congenital in the western region of Paraná, Brazil. Rev Bras Ginecol Obstet 2012; 34(2): 63-8.
[PMID: 22437764]

[23]  Sparkes AH. Toxoplasmosis en el gato y en el hombre. Buenos Aires, Argentina: Congresso de la Asociación Mundial de Medicina Veterinaria de Pequeños Animales 1998; pp. 415-7.

[24]  Robert-Gangneux F, Dardé ML. Epidemiology of and diagnostic strategies for toxoplasmosis. Clin Microbiol Rev 2012; 25(2): 264-96.
[http://dx.doi.org/10.1128/CMR.05013-11] [PMID: 22491772]

[25]  Dunn D, Wallon M, Peyron F, Petersen E, Peckham C, Gilbert R. Mother-to-child transmission of toxoplasmosis: risk estimates for clinical counselling. Lancet 1999; 353(9167): 1829-33.
[http://dx.doi.org/10.1016/S0140-6736(98)08220-8] [PMID: 10359407]

[26]  Abbasi M, Kowalewska-Grochowska K, Bahar MA, Kilani RT, Winkler-Lowen B, Guilbert LJ. Infection of placental trophoblasts by *Toxoplasma gondii*. J Infect Dis 2003; 188(4): 608-16.
[http://dx.doi.org/10.1086/377132] [PMID: 12898451]

[27]  Desmonts G, Couvreur J. Congenital toxoplasmosis. A prospective study of 378 pregnancies. N Engl J Med 1974; 290(20): 1110-6.
[http://dx.doi.org/10.1056/NEJM197405162902003] [PMID: 4821174]

[28]  Hohlfeld P, Daffos F, Costa J-M, Thulliez P, Forestier F, Vidaud M. Prenatal diagnosis of congenital toxoplasmosis with a polymerase-chain-reaction test on amniotic fluid. N Engl J Med 1994; 331(11): 695-9.
[http://dx.doi.org/10.1056/NEJM199409153311102] [PMID: 8058075]

[29]  Remington J, McLeod R, Desmonts G. Toxoplasmosis.Infectious diseases of the fetus and newborn infant. 6th ed. Philadelphia: Elsevier Saunders 2006; pp. 947-1091.
[http://dx.doi.org/10.1016/B0-72-160537-0/50033-5]

[30]  Pinard JA, Leslie NS, Irvine PJ. Maternal serologic screening for toxoplasmosis. J Midwifery Womens Health 2003; 48(5): 308-16.
[http://dx.doi.org/10.1016/S1526-9523(03)00279-4] [PMID: 14526343]

[31]  Frenkel JK. Toxoplasmose.Tratado de Infectologia. São Paulo: Guanabara Koogan 2002; pp. 1310-24.

[32]  Sabin AB. Toxoplasmosis: recently recognized disease. Adv Pediatr 1942; 1: 1-54.

[33]  Olariu TR, Remington JS, McLeod R, Alam A, Montoya JG. Severe congenital toxoplasmosis in the

United States: clinical and serologic findings in untreated infants. Pediatr Infect Dis J 2011; 30(12): 1056-61.
[http://dx.doi.org/10.1097/INF.0b013e3182343096] [PMID: 21956696]

[34] Wilson CB, Remington JS, Stagno S, Reynolds DW. Development of adverse sequelae in children born with subclinical congenital Toxoplasma infection. Pediatrics 1980; 66(5): 767-74.
[PMID: 7432882]

[35] Amendoeira MR. LF. C-C. Uma breve revisão sobre toxoplasmose na gestação. Sci Med 2010; 20(1): 113-9.

[36] Cook AJ, Gilbert RE, Buffolano W, *et al.* European Research Network on Congenital Toxoplasmosis. Sources of toxoplasma infection in pregnant women: European multicentre case-control study. BMJ 2000; 321(7254): 142-7.
[http://dx.doi.org/10.1136/bmj.321.7254.142] [PMID: 10894691]

[37] Silveira C, Ferreira R, Muccioli C, Nussenblatt R, Belfort R Jr. Toxoplasmosis transmitted to a newborn from the mother infected 20 years earlier. Am J Ophthalmol 2003; 136(2): 370-1.
[http://dx.doi.org/10.1016/S0002-9394(03)00191-0] [PMID: 12888070]

[38] Kodjikian L, Hoigne I, Adam O, *et al.* Vertical transmission of toxoplasmosis from a chronically infected immunocompetent woman. Pediatr Infect Dis J 2004; 23(3): 272-4.
[http://dx.doi.org/10.1097/01.inf.0000115949.12206.69] [PMID: 15014310]

[39] Lebas F, Ducrocq S, Mucignat V, *et al.* Congenital toxoplasmosis: a new case of infection during pregnancy in an previously immunized and immunocompetent woman. Arch Pediatr 2004; 11(8): 926-8. [Congenital toxoplasmosis: a new case of infection during pregnancy in an previously immunized and immunocompetent woman].
[http://dx.doi.org/10.1016/j.arcped.2004.04.017] [PMID: 15288083]

[40] Elbez-Rubinstein A, Ajzenberg D, Dardé ML, *et al.* Congenital toxoplasmosis and reinfection during pregnancy: case report, strain characterization, experimental model of reinfection, and review. J Infect Dis 2009; 199(2): 280-5.
[http://dx.doi.org/10.1086/595793] [PMID: 19032062]

[41] Robert-Gangneux F. It is not only the cat that did it: how to prevent and treat congenital toxoplasmosis. J Infect 2014; 68 (Suppl. 1): S125-33.
[http://dx.doi.org/10.1016/j.jinf.2013.09.023] [PMID: 24119928]

[42] Bachmeyer C, Mouchnino G, Thulliez P, Blum L. Congenital toxoplasmosis from an HIV-infected woman as a result of reactivation. J Infect 2006; 52(2): e55-7.
[http://dx.doi.org/10.1016/j.jinf.2005.05.004] [PMID: 16043225]

[43] Lindsay DS, Dubey JP. *Toxoplasma gondii*: the changing paradigm of congenital toxoplasmosis. Parasitology 2011; 138(14): 1829-31.
[http://dx.doi.org/10.1017/S0031182011001478] [PMID: 21902872]

[44] Marty P, Le Fichoux Y, Deville A, Forest H. Congenital toxoplasmosis and preconceptional maternal ganglionic toxoplasmosis. Presse Med 1991; 20(8): 387.
[PMID: 1826773]

[45] Dardé ML, Bouteille B, Pestre-Alexandre M. Isoenzyme analysis of 35 *Toxoplasma gondii* isolates and the biological and epidemiological implications. J Parasitol 1992; 78(5): 786-94.
[http://dx.doi.org/10.2307/3283305] [PMID: 1403418]

[46] Ajzenberg D, Cogné N, Paris L, *et al.* Genotype of 86 *Toxoplasma gondii* isolates associated with human congenital toxoplasmosis, and correlation with clinical findings. J Infect Dis 2002; 186(5): 684-9.
[http://dx.doi.org/10.1086/342663] [PMID: 12195356]

[47] Ajzenberg D, Bañuls AL, Su C, *et al.* Genetic diversity, clonality and sexuality in *Toxoplasma gondii*. Int J Parasitol 2004; 34(10): 1185-96.

[http://dx.doi.org/10.1016/j.ijpara.2004.06.007] [PMID: 15380690]

[48]    Dubey JP, Sundar N, Pineda N, *et al.* Biologic and genetic characteristics of *Toxoplasma gondii* isolates in free-range chickens from Nicaragua, Central America. Vet Parasitol 2006; 142(1-2): 47-53. [http://dx.doi.org/10.1016/j.vetpar.2006.06.016] [PMID: 16876324]

[49]    Dubey JP, Applewhaite L, Sundar N, Velmurugan GV, Bandini LA, Kwok OC, *et al.* Molecular and biological characterization of *Toxoplasma gondii* isolates from free-range chickens from Guyana, South America, identified several unique and common parasite genotypes. Parasitology 2007;134 [Pt 11 ]:1559-65.

[50]    Dubey JP, Gennari SM, Sundar N, *et al.* Diverse and atypical genotypes identified in *Toxoplasma gondii* from dogs in São Paulo, Brazil. J Parasitol 2007; 93(1): 60-4. [http://dx.doi.org/10.1645/GE-972R.1] [PMID: 17436942]

[51]    Pena HF, Gennari SM, Dubey JP, Su C. Population structure and mouse-virulence of *Toxoplasma gondii* in Brazil. Int J Parasitol 2008; 38(5): 561-9. [http://dx.doi.org/10.1016/j.ijpara.2007.09.004] [PMID: 17963770]

[52]    Aubert D, Ajzenberg D, Richomme C, *et al.* Molecular and biological characteristics of *Toxoplasma gondii* isolates from wildlife in France. Vet Parasitol 2010; 171(3-4): 346-9. [http://dx.doi.org/10.1016/j.vetpar.2010.03.033] [PMID: 20417034]

[53]    Beck HP, Blake D, Dardé ML, *et al.* Molecular approaches to diversity of populations of apicomplexan parasites. Int J Parasitol 2009; 39(2): 175-89. [http://dx.doi.org/10.1016/j.ijpara.2008.10.001] [PMID: 18983997]

[54]    Pomares C, Ajzenberg D, Bornard L, *et al.* Toxoplasmosis and horse meat, France. Emerg Infect Dis 2011; 17(7): 1327-8. [http://dx.doi.org/10.3201/eid1707.101642] [PMID: 21762609]

[55]    Howe DK, Sibley LD. *Toxoplasma gondii* comprises three clonal lineages: correlation of parasite genotype with human disease. J Infect Dis 1995; 172(6): 1561-6. [http://dx.doi.org/10.1093/infdis/172.6.1561] [PMID: 7594717]

[56]    Khan A, Dubey JP, Su C, Ajioka JW, Rosenthal BM, Sibley LD. Genetic analyses of atypical *Toxoplasma gondii* strains reveal a fourth clonal lineage in North America. Int J Parasitol 2011; 41(6): 645-55. [http://dx.doi.org/10.1016/j.ijpara.2011.01.005] [PMID: 21320505]

[57]    Carme B, Bissuel F, Ajzenberg D, *et al.* Severe acquired toxoplasmosis in immunocompetent adult patients in French Guiana. J Clin Microbiol 2002; 40(11): 4037-44. [http://dx.doi.org/10.1128/JCM.40.11.4037-4044.2002] [PMID: 12409371]

[58]    Gilbert RE, Freeman K, Lago EG, *et al.* European Multicentre Study on Congenital Toxoplasmosis (EMSCOT). Ocular sequelae of congenital toxoplasmosis in Brazil compared with Europe. PLoS Negl Trop Dis 2008; 2(8): e277. [http://dx.doi.org/10.1371/journal.pntd.0000277] [PMID: 18698419]

[59]    Jones J, Lopez A, Wilson M. Congenital toxoplasmosis. Am Fam Physician 2003; 67(10): 2131-8. [PMID: 12776962]

[60]    Gras L, Gilbert RE, Wallon M, Peyron F, Cortina-Borja M. Duration of the IgM response in women acquiring *Toxoplasma gondii* during pregnancy: implications for clinical practice and cross-sectional incidence studies. Epidemiol Infect 2004; 132(3): 541-8. [http://dx.doi.org/10.1017/S0950268803001948] [PMID: 15188723]

[61]    Montoya JG, Rosso F. Diagnosis and management of toxoplasmosis. Clin Perinatol 2005; 32(3): 705-26. [http://dx.doi.org/10.1016/j.clp.2005.04.011] [PMID: 16085028]

[62]    Nascimento FS, Suzuki LA, Rossi CL. Assessment of the value of detecting specific IgA antibodies for the diagnosis of a recently acquired primary *Toxoplasma* infection. Prenat Diagn 2008; 28(8): 749-

52.
[http://dx.doi.org/10.1002/pd.2052] [PMID: 18618923]

[63]     Remington JS, McLeod R, Wilson CB, Desmonts G. Toxoplasmosis.Infectious Diseases of the Fetus
          and Newborn. Philadelphia: W.B. Saunders 2011; pp. 918-1041. [Seventh Edition ]
          [http://dx.doi.org/10.1016/B978-1-4160-6400-8.00031-6]

[64]     Franck J, Garin YJ, Dumon H. LDBio-Toxo II immunoglobulin G Western blot confirmatory test for
          anti-toxoplasma antibody detection. J Clin Microbiol 2008; 46(7): 2334-8.
          [http://dx.doi.org/10.1128/JCM.00182-08] [PMID: 18480220]

[65]     Dhakal R, Gajurel K, Pomares C, Talucod J, Press CJ, Montoya JG. Significance of a Positive
          *Toxoplasma* Immunoglobulin M Test Result in the United States. J Clin Microbiol 2015; 53(11):
          3601-5.
          [http://dx.doi.org/10.1128/JCM.01663-15] [PMID: 26354818]

[66]     Lappalainen M, Koskela P, Koskiniemi M, *et al.* Toxoplasmosis acquired during pregnancy: improved
          serodiagnosis based on avidity of IgG. J Infect Dis 1993; 167(3): 691-7.
          [http://dx.doi.org/10.1093/infdis/167.3.691] [PMID: 8440939]

[67]     Barina R, Bianchi MO, Camargo MM, Silva EA, Marba ST. Toxoplasmose: um diagnóstico difícil
          com testes sorológicos automatizados. Annual Meeting Fetal Medicine and Surgery Society;
          Nantucker. MA, USA2000.

[68]     Montoya JG, Liesenfeld O, Kinney S, Press C, Remington JS. VIDAS test for avidity of Toxoplasma-
          specific immunoglobulin G for confirmatory testing of pregnant women. J Clin Microbiol 2002; 40(7):
          2504-8.

[69]     Liesenfeld O, Montoya JG, Kinney S, Press C, Remington JS. Effect of testing for IgG avidity in the
          diagnosis of *Toxoplasma gondii* infection in pregnant women: experience in a US reference laboratory.
          J Infect Dis 2001; 183(8): 1248-53.
          [http://dx.doi.org/10.1086/319672] [PMID: 11262207]

[70]     Lebech M, Andersen O, Christensen NC, *et al.* Danish Congenital Toxoplasmosis Study Group.
          Feasibility of neonatal screening for toxoplasma infection in the absence of prenatal treatment. Lancet
          1999; 353(9167): 1834-7.
          [http://dx.doi.org/10.1016/S0140-6736(98)11281-3] [PMID: 10359408]

[71]     Candolfi E, Pastor R, Huber R, Filisetti D, Villard O. IgG avidity assay firms up the diagnosis of acute
          toxoplasmosis on the first serum sample in immunocompetent pregnant women. Diagn Microbiol
          Infect Dis 2007; 58(1): 83-8.
          [http://dx.doi.org/10.1016/j.diagmicrobio.2006.12.010] [PMID: 17368807]

[72]     Roberts F, Mets MB, Ferguson DJ, *et al.* Histopathological features of ocular toxoplasmosis in the
          fetus and infant. Arch Ophthalmol 2001; 119(1): 51-8.
          [PMID: 11146726]

[73]     Carellos EV, Andrade GM, Aguiar RA. Evaluation of prenatal screening for toxoplasmosis in Belo
          Horizonte, Minas Gerais State, Brazil: a cross-sectional study of postpartum women in two maternity
          hospitals. Cad Saude Publica 2008; 24(2): 391-401.
          [http://dx.doi.org/10.1590/S0102-311X2008000200018] [PMID: 18278286]

[74]     Lefevre-Pettazzoni M, Bissery A, Wallon M, Cozon G, Peyron F, Rabilloud M. Impact of spiramycin
          treatment and gestational age on maturation of *Toxoplasma gondii* immunoglobulin G avidity in
          pregnant women. Clin Vaccine Immunol 2007; 14(3): 239-43.
          [http://dx.doi.org/10.1128/CVI.00311-06] [PMID: 17202303]

[75]     Reis MM, Tessaro MM, D'Azevedo PA. *Toxoplasma*-IgM and IgG-avidity in single samples from
          areas with a high infection rate can determine the risk of mother-to-child transmission. Rev Inst Med
          Trop São Paulo 2006; 48(2): 93-8.
          [http://dx.doi.org/10.1590/S0036-46652006000200007] [PMID: 16699631]

[76]    Giraldo M, Portela RW, Snege M, *et al.* Immunoglobulin M (IgM)-glycoinositolphospholipid enzyme-linked immunosorbent assay: an immunoenzymatic assay for discrimination between patients with acute toxoplasmosis and those with persistent parasite-specific IgM antibodies. J Clin Microbiol 2002; 40(4): 1400-5.
[http://dx.doi.org/10.1128/JCM.40.4.1400-1405.2002] [PMID: 11923364]

[77]    Beghetto E, Buffolano W, Spadoni A, *et al.* Use of an immunoglobulin G avidity assay based on recombinant antigens for diagnosis of primary *Toxoplasma gondii* infection during pregnancy. J Clin Microbiol 2003; 41(12): 5414-8.
[http://dx.doi.org/10.1128/JCM.41.12.5414-5418.2003] [PMID: 14662919]

[78]    Kotresha D, Noordin R. Recombinant proteins in the diagnosis of toxoplasmosis. APMIS 2010; 118(8): 529-42.
[PMID: 20666734]

[79]    Pietkiewicz H, Hiszczyńska-Sawicka E, Kur J, *et al.* Usefulness of *Toxoplasma gondii* recombinant antigens (GRA1, GRA7 and SAG1) in an immunoglobulin G avidity test for the serodiagnosis of toxoplasmosis. Parasitol Res 2007; 100(2): 333-7.
[http://dx.doi.org/10.1007/s00436-006-0265-1] [PMID: 16896649]

[80]    Bessières M-H, Chemla C, Cimon B, Marty P, Gay-Andrieu F, Pellouv H, *et al.* Les difficultés d'interprétation de la sérologie de la toxoplasmose. Revue Francophone des Laboratoires 2006; 2006(383): 43-9.
[http://dx.doi.org/10.1016/S1773-035X(06)80229-7]

[81]    Foulon W, Pinon JM, Stray-Pedersen B, *et al.* Prenatal diagnosis of congenital toxoplasmosis: a multicenter evaluation of different diagnostic parameters. Am J Obstet Gynecol 1999; 181(4): 843-7.
[http://dx.doi.org/10.1016/S0002-9378(99)70311-X] [PMID: 10521739]

[82]    Abboud P, Villena I, Chemla C, *et al.* Screening for congenital toxoplasmosis: pregnancy outcome after prenatal diagnosis in 211 cases. J Gynecol Obstet Biol Reprod (Paris) 1997; 26(1): 40-6.
[PMID: 9091543]

[83]    Dorangeon P, Fay R, Marx-Chemla C, *et al.* Transplacental passage of the pyrimethamine-sulfadoxine combination in the prenatal treatment of congenital toxoplasmosis. Presse Med 1990; 19(44): 2036.
[PMID: 2148622]

[84]    Hohlfeld P, Daffos F, Thulliez P, *et al.* Fetal toxoplasmosis: outcome of pregnancy and infant follow-up after in utero treatment. J Pediatr 1989; 115(5 Pt 1): 765-9.
[http://dx.doi.org/10.1016/S0022-3476(89)80660-2] [PMID: 2681638]

[85]    Bastien P. Molecular diagnosis of toxoplasmosis. Trans R Soc Trop Med Hyg 2002; 96 (Suppl. 1): S205-15.
[http://dx.doi.org/10.1016/S0035-9203(02)90078-7] [PMID: 12055840]

[86]    Daffos F, Forestier F, Capella-Pavlovsky M, *et al.* Prenatal management of 746 pregnancies at risk for congenital toxoplasmosis. N Engl J Med 1988; 318(5): 271-5.
[http://dx.doi.org/10.1056/NEJM198802043180502] [PMID: 3336419]

[87]    Couto JC, Melo RN, Rodrigues MV, Leite JM. Diagnóstico pré-natal e tratamento da toxoplasmose na gestação. Femina 2003; 31: 85-90.

[88]    Grover CM, Thulliez P, Remington JS, Boothroyd JC. Rapid prenatal diagnosis of congenital *Toxoplasma* infection by using polymerase chain reaction and amniotic fluid. J Clin Microbiol 1990; 28(10): 2297-301.
[PMID: 2229355]

[89]    Desmonts G, Daffos F, Forestier F, Capella-Pavlovsky M, Thulliez P, Chartier M. Prenatal diagnosis of congenital toxoplasmosis. Lancet 1985; 1(8427): 500-4.
[http://dx.doi.org/10.1016/S0140-6736(85)92096-3] [PMID: 2857860]

[90]    Homan WL, Vercammen M, De Braekeleer J, Verschueren H. Identification of a 200- to 300-fold

repetitive 529 bp DNA fragment in *Toxoplasma gondii*, and its use for diagnostic and quantitative PCR. Int J Parasitol 2000; 30(1): 69-75.
[http://dx.doi.org/10.1016/S0020-7519(99)00170-8] [PMID: 10675747]

[91]    Romand S, Chosson M, Franck J, *et al.* Usefulness of quantitative polymerase chain reaction in amniotic fluid as early prognostic marker of fetal infection with *Toxoplasma gondii*. Am J Obstet Gynecol 2004; 190(3): 797-802.
[http://dx.doi.org/10.1016/j.ajog.2003.09.039] [PMID: 15042017]

[92]    Vidigal PV, Santos DV, Castro FC, Couto JC, Vitor RW, Brasileiro Filho G. Prenatal toxoplasmosis diagnosis from amniotic fluid by PCR. Rev Soc Bras Med Trop 2002; 35(1): 1-6.
[http://dx.doi.org/10.1590/S0037-86822002000100001] [PMID: 11873253]

[93]    Robert-Gangneux F, Gavinet MF, Ancelle T, Raymond J, Tourte-Schaefer C, Dupouy-Camet J. Value of prenatal diagnosis and early postnatal diagnosis of congenital toxoplasmosis: retrospective study of 110 cases. J Clin Microbiol 1999; 37(9): 2893-8.
[PMID: 10449471]

[94]    Pelloux H, Guy E, Angelici MC, *et al.* A second European collaborative study on polymerase chain reaction for *Toxoplasma gondii*, involving 15 teams. FEMS Microbiol Lett 1998; 165(2): 231-7.
[http://dx.doi.org/10.1111/j.1574-6968.1998.tb13151.x] [PMID: 9742693]

[95]    Kaiser K, Van Loon AM, Pelloux H, *et al.* Multicenter proficiency study for detection of *Toxoplasma gondii* in amniotic fluid by nucleic acid amplification methods. Clin Chim Acta 2007; 375(1-2): 99-103.
[http://dx.doi.org/10.1016/j.cca.2006.06.016] [PMID: 16860303]

[96]    Maubon D, Brenier-Pinchart MP, Fricker-Hidalgo H, Pelloux H. Real-time PCR in the diagnosis of toxoplasmosis: the way to standardisation?. Pathol Biol (Paris) 2007; 55(6): 304-11.
[http://dx.doi.org/10.1016/j.patbio.2006.11.001] [PMID: 17303349]

[97]    Yera H, Filisetti D, Bastien P, Ancelle T, Thulliez P, Delhaes L. Multicenter comparative evaluation of five commercial methods for toxoplasma DNA extraction from amniotic fluid. J Clin Microbiol 2009; 47(12): 3881-6.
[http://dx.doi.org/10.1128/JCM.01164-09] [PMID: 19846633]

[98]    Bastien P, Jumas-Bilak E, Varlet-Marie E, Marty P. ANOFEL Toxoplasma-PCR Quality Control Group. Three years of multi-laboratory external quality control for the molecular detection of *Toxoplasma gondii* in amniotic fluid in France. Clin Microbiol Infect 2007; 13(4): 430-3.
[http://dx.doi.org/10.1111/j.1469-0691.2006.01642.x] [PMID: 17359328]

[99]    Sterkers Y, Varlet-Marie E, Cassaing S, *et al.* Multicentric comparative analytical performance study for molecular detection of low amounts of *Toxoplasma gondii* from simulated specimens. J Clin Microbiol 2010; 48(9): 3216-22.
[http://dx.doi.org/10.1128/JCM.02500-09] [PMID: 20610670]

[100]   Wallon M, Franck J, Thulliez P, *et al.* Accuracy of real-time polymerase chain reaction for *Toxoplasma gondii* in amniotic fluid. Obstet Gynecol 2010; 115(4): 727-33.
[http://dx.doi.org/10.1097/AOG.0b013e3181d57b09] [PMID: 20308831]

[101]   Romand S, Wallon M, Franck J, Thulliez P, Peyron F, Dumon H. Prenatal diagnosis using polymerase chain reaction on amniotic fluid for congenital toxoplasmosis. Obstet Gynecol 2001; 97(2): 296-300.
[PMID: 11165598]

[102]   Bessières MH, Cassaing S, Berrebi A, Séguéla JP. Apport des techniques de biologie moléculaire dans le diagnostic prénatal de la toxoplasmose congénitale. Immunol Anal Biol Spec 2002; 17(6): 358-62.
[http://dx.doi.org/10.1016/S0923-2532(02)01224-3]

[103]   Castro FC, Castro MJBV, Cabral ACV, Brasileiro Filho G. Comparação dos métodos para diagnóstico da toxoplasmose congênita. Rev Bras Ginecol Obstet 2001; 23: 277-82.
[http://dx.doi.org/10.1590/S0100-72032001000500002]

[104] Filisetti D, Gorcii M, Pernot-Marino E, Villard O, Candolfi E. Diagnosis of congenital toxoplasmosis: comparison of targets for detection of *Toxoplasma gondii* by PCR. J Clin Microbiol 2003; 41(10): 4826-8.
[http://dx.doi.org/10.1128/JCM.41.10.4826-4828.2003] [PMID: 14532233]

[105] Montoya JG, Liesenfeld O. Toxoplasmosis. Lancet 2004; 363(9425): 1965-76.

[106] Wallon M, Peyron F, Cornu C, *et al.* Congenital toxoplasma infection: monthly prenatal screening decreases transmission rate and improves clinical outcome at age 3 years. Clin Infect Dis 2013; 56(9): 1223-31.
[http://dx.doi.org/10.1093/cid/cit032] [PMID: 23362291]

[107] Gilbert R, Gras L. European Multicentre Study on Congenital Toxoplasmosis. Effect of timing and type of treatment on the risk of mother to child transmission of *Toxoplasma gondii*. BJOG 2003; 110(2): 112-20.
[http://dx.doi.org/10.1046/j.1471-0528.2003.02325.x] [PMID: 12618153]

[108] Thiébaut R, Leproust S, Chêne G, Gilbert R. SYROCOT (Systematic Review on Congenital Toxoplasmosis) study group. Effectiveness of prenatal treatment for congenital toxoplasmosis: a meta-analysis of individual patients' data. Lancet 2007; 369(9556): 115-22.
[http://dx.doi.org/10.1016/S0140-6736(07)60072-5] [PMID: 17223474]

[109] Galanakis E, Manoura A, Antoniou M, *et al.* Outcome of toxoplasmosis acquired during pregnancy following treatment in both pregnancy and early infancy. Fetal Diagn Ther 2007; 22(6): 444-8.
[http://dx.doi.org/10.1159/000106352] [PMID: 17652934]

[110] Aspöck H, Pollak A. Prevention of prenatal toxoplasmosis by serological screening of pregnant women in Austria. Scand J Infect Dis Suppl 1992; 84: 32-7.
[PMID: 1290071]

[111] Prusa AR, Kasper DC, Pollak A, Olischar M, Gleiss A, Hayde M. Amniocentesis for the detection of congenital toxoplasmosis: results from the nationwide Austrian prenatal screening program. Clin Microbiol Infect 2015; 21(2): 191-191.e1-8.

[112] Khoshnood B, De Vigan C, Goffinet F, Leroy V. Prenatal screening and diagnosis of congenital toxoplasmosis: a review of safety issues and psychological consequences for women who undergo screening. Prenat Diagn 2007; 27(5): 395-403.
[http://dx.doi.org/10.1002/pd.1715] [PMID: 17380472]

[113] Garin JP, Pellerat J, Maillard , Woehrle R, Hezez . Theoretical bases of the prevention by spiramycin of congenital toxoplasmosis in pregnant women. Presse Med 1968; 76(48): 2266.
[PMID: 5720932]

[114] Wallon M, Liou C, Garner P, Peyron F. Congenital toxoplasmosis: systematic review of evidence of efficacy of treatment in pregnancy. BMJ 1999; 318(7197): 1511-4.
[http://dx.doi.org/10.1136/bmj.318.7197.1511] [PMID: 10356003]

[115] Cortina-Borja M, Tan HK, Wallon M, *et al.* European Multicentre Study on Congenital Toxoplasmosis (EMSCOT). Prenatal treatment for serious neurological sequelae of congenital toxoplasmosis: an observational prospective cohort study. PLoS Med 2010; 7(10): 7. [10 ].
[http://dx.doi.org/10.1371/journal.pmed.1000351] [PMID: 20967235]

[116] Gras L, Wallon M, Pollak A, *et al.* European Multicenter Study on Congenital Toxoplasmosis. Association between prenatal treatment and clinical manifestations of congenital toxoplasmosis in infancy: a cohort study in 13 European centres. Acta Paediatr 2005; 94(12): 1721-31.
[http://dx.doi.org/10.1080/08035250500251999] [PMID: 16421031]

[117] Vasconcelos-Santos DV, Machado Azevedo DO, Campos WR, *et al.* Congenital toxoplasmosis in southeastern Brazil: results of early ophthalmologic examination of a large cohort of neonates. Ophthalmology 2009; 116(11): 2199-2205.e1.

[118] Dubey JP. Duration of immunity to shedding of *Toxoplasma gondii* oocysts by cats. J Parasitol 1995;

81(3): 410-5.
[http://dx.doi.org/10.2307/3283823] [PMID: 7776126]

[119] Tenter AM, Heckeroth AR, Weiss LM. *Toxoplasma gondii*: from animals to humans. Int J Parasitol 2000; 30(12-13): 1217-58.
[http://dx.doi.org/10.1016/S0020-7519(00)00124-7] [PMID: 11113252]

[120] de Moura L, Bahia-Oliveira LM, Wada MY, *et al.* Waterborne toxoplasmosis, Brazil, from field to gene. Emerg Infect Dis 2006; 12(2): 326-9.
[http://dx.doi.org/10.3201/eid1202.041115] [PMID: 16494765]

[121] Heukelbach J, Meyer-Cirkel V, Moura RC, *et al.* Waterborne toxoplasmosis, northeastern Brazil. Emerg Infect Dis 2007; 13(2): 287-9.
[http://dx.doi.org/10.3201/eid1302.060686] [PMID: 17479893]

[122] Palanisamy M, Madhavan B, Balasundaram MB, Andavar R, Venkatapathy N. Outbreak of ocular toxoplasmosis in Coimbatore, India. Indian J Ophthalmol 2006; 54(2): 129-31.
[http://dx.doi.org/10.4103/0301-4738.25839] [PMID: 16770035]

[123] Boyer K, Hill D, Mui E, *et al.* Toxoplasmosis Study Group. Unrecognized ingestion of *Toxoplasma gondii* oocysts leads to congenital toxoplasmosis and causes epidemics in North America. Clin Infect Dis 2011; 53(11): 1081-9.
[http://dx.doi.org/10.1093/cid/cir667] [PMID: 22021924]

[124] Bowie WR, King AS, Werker DH, *et al.* Outbreak of toxoplasmosis associated with municipal drinking water. The BC Toxoplasma Investigation Team. Lancet 1997; 350(9072): 173-7.

[125] Gollub EL, Leroy V, Gilbert R, Chêne G, Wallon M. European Toxoprevention Study Group (EUROTOXO). Effectiveness of health education on *Toxoplasma*-related knowledge, behaviour, and risk of seroconversion in pregnancy. Eur J Obstet Gynecol Reprod Biol 2008; 136(2): 137-45.
[http://dx.doi.org/10.1016/j.ejogrb.2007.09.010] [PMID: 17977641]

[126] Foulon W, Naessens A, Derde MP. Evaluation of the possibilities for preventing congenital toxoplasmosis. Am J Perinatol 1994; 11(1): 57-62.
[http://dx.doi.org/10.1055/s-2007-994537] [PMID: 8155214]

[127] Pawlowski ZS, Gromadecka-Sutkiewicz M, Skommer J, *et al.* Impact of health education on knowledge and prevention behavior for congenital toxoplasmosis: the experience in Poznań, Poland. Health Educ Res 2001; 16(4): 493-502.
[http://dx.doi.org/10.1093/her/16.4.493] [PMID: 11525395]

[128] Conyn-van Spaedonck MA, van Knapen F. Choices in preventive strategies: experience with the prevention of congenital toxoplasmosis in The Netherlands. Scand J Infect Dis Suppl 1992; 84: 51-8.
[PMID: 1290075]

[129] Kravetz JD, Federman DG. Toxoplasmosis in pregnancy. Am J Med 2005; 118(3): 212-6.
[http://dx.doi.org/10.1016/j.amjmed.2004.08.023] [PMID: 15745715]

[130] Paul M, Petersen E, Pawlowski ZS, Szczapa J. Neonatal screening for congenital toxoplasmosis in the Poznań region of Poland by analysis of *Toxoplasma gondii*-specific IgM antibodies eluted from filter paper blood spots. Pediatr Infect Dis J 2000; 19(1): 30-6.
[http://dx.doi.org/10.1097/00006454-200001000-00007] [PMID: 10643847]

[131] Boyer KM, Holfels E, Roizen N, *et al.* Toxoplasmosis Study Group. Risk factors for *Toxoplasma gondii* infection in mothers of infants with congenital toxoplasmosis: Implications for prenatal management and screening. Am J Obstet Gynecol 2005; 192(2): 564-71.
[http://dx.doi.org/10.1016/j.ajog.2004.07.031] [PMID: 15696004]

[132] Guerina NG, Hsu HW, Meissner HC, *et al.* The New England Regional Toxoplasma Working Group. Neonatal serologic screening and early treatment for congenital *Toxoplasma gondii* infection. N Engl J Med 1994; 330(26): 1858-63.
[http://dx.doi.org/10.1056/NEJM199406303302604] [PMID: 7818637]

[133]  Capobiango JD, Breganó RM, Navarro IT, *et al.* Congenital toxoplasmosis in a reference center of Paraná, Southern Brazil. Braz J Infect Dis 2014; 18(4): 364-71.
[http://dx.doi.org/10.1016/j.bjid.2013.11.009] [PMID: 24662141]

[134]  Gilbert RE, Thalib L, Tan HK, Paul M, Wallon M, Petersen E. European Multicentre Study on Congenital Toxoplasmosis. Screening for congenital toxoplasmosis: accuracy of immunoglobulin M and immunoglobulin A tests after birth. J Med Screen 2007; 14(1): 8-13.
[http://dx.doi.org/10.1258/096914107780154440] [PMID: 17362565]

[135]  Bessières MH, Berrebi A, Rolland M, *et al.* Neonatal screening for congenital toxoplasmosis in a cohort of 165 women infected during pregnancy and influence of in utero treatment on the results of neonatal tests. Eur J Obstet Gynecol Reprod Biol 2001; 94(1): 37-45.
[http://dx.doi.org/10.1016/S0301-2115(00)00300-6] [PMID: 11134824]

[136]  Lago EG, Neto EC, Melamed J, *et al.* Congenital toxoplasmosis: late pregnancy infections detected by neonatal screening and maternal serological testing at delivery. Paediatr Perinat Epidemiol 2007; 21(6): 525-31.
[http://dx.doi.org/10.1111/j.1365-3016.2007.00869.x] [PMID: 17937738]

[137]  Sensini A. *Toxoplasma gondii* infection in pregnancy: opportunities and pitfalls of serological diagnosis. Clin Microbiol Infect 2006; 12(6): 504-12.

[138]  Gross U, Luder CG, Hendgen V, *et al.* Comparative immunoglobulin G antibody profiles between mother and child (CGMC test) for early diagnosis of congenital toxoplasmosis. J Clin Microbiol 2000; 38(10): 3619-22.

[139]  Pinon JM, Dumon H, Chemla C, *et al.* Strategy for diagnosis of congenital toxoplasmosis: evaluation of methods comparing mothers and newborns and standard methods for postnatal detection of immunoglobulin G, M, and A antibodies. J Clin Microbiol 2001; 39(6): 2267-71.
[http://dx.doi.org/10.1128/JCM.39.6.2267-2271.2001] [PMID: 11376068]

[140]  Remington JS, Araujo FG, Desmonts G. Recognition of different *Toxoplasma* antigens by IgM and IgG antibodies in mothers and their congenitally infected newborns. J Infect Dis 1985; 152(5): 1020-4.
[http://dx.doi.org/10.1093/infdis/152.5.1020] [PMID: 2413141]

[141]  Tissot Dupont D, Fricker-Hidalgo H, Brenier-Pinchart MP, Bost-Bru C, Ambroise-Thomas P, Pelloux H. Usefulness of Western blot in serological follow-up of newborns suspected of congenital toxoplasmosis. Eur J Clin Microbiol Infect Dis 2003; 22(2): 122-5.
[PMID: 12627289]

[142]  Capobiango JD, Monica TC, Ferreira FP, *et al.* Evaluation of the Western blotting method for the diagnosis of congenital toxoplasmosis. J Pediatr 2016; 92(6): 616-23.

[143]  Machado AS, Andrade GM, Januário JN, *et al.* IgG and IgM western blot assay for diagnosis of congenital toxoplasmosis. Mem Inst Oswaldo Cruz 2010; 105(6): 757-61.
[http://dx.doi.org/10.1590/S0074-02762010000600005] [PMID: 20944989]

[144]  Rilling V, Dietz K, Krczal D, Knotek F, Enders G. Evaluation of a commercial IgG/IgM Western blot assay for early postnatal diagnosis of congenital toxoplasmosis. Eur J Clin Microbiol Infect Dis 2003; 22(3): 174-80.

[145]  Buffolano W. Congenital toxoplasmosis: the state of the art. Parassitologia 2008; 50(1-2): 37-43.

[146]  Antoniou M, Tzouvali H, Sifakis S, *et al.* Incidence of toxoplasmosis in 5532 pregnant women in Crete, Greece: management of 185 cases at risk. Eur J Obstet Gynecol Reprod Biol 2004; 117(2): 138-43.
[http://dx.doi.org/10.1016/j.ejogrb.2004.03.001] [PMID: 15541847]

[147]  Parmley SF, Goebel FD, Remington JS. Detection of *Toxoplasma gondii* in cerebrospinal fluid from AIDS patients by polymerase chain reaction. J Clin Microbiol 1992; 30(11): 3000-2.
[PMID: 1452673]

[148]   Reischl U, Bretagne S, Krüger D, Ernault P, Costa JM. Comparison of two DNA targets for the diagnosis of Toxoplasmosis by real-time PCR using fluorescence resonance energy transfer hybridization probes. BMC Infect Dis 2003; 3: 7.
[http://dx.doi.org/10.1186/1471-2334-3-7] [PMID: 12729464]

[149]   Costa JG, Carneiro AC, Tavares AT, *et al.* Real-time PCR as a prognostic tool for human congenital toxoplasmosis. J Clin Microbiol 2013; 51(8): 2766-8.

[150]   McLeod R, Boyer K, Karrison T, *et al.* Toxoplasmosis Study Group. Outcome of treatment for congenital toxoplasmosis, 1981-2004: the National Collaborative Chicago-Based, Congenital Toxoplasmosis Study. Clin Infect Dis 2006; 42(10): 1383-94.
[http://dx.doi.org/10.1086/501360] [PMID: 16619149]

[151]   McLeod R, Kieffer F, Sautter M, Hosten T, Pelloux H. Why prevent, diagnose and treat congenital toxoplasmosis? Mem Inst Oswaldo Cruz 2009; 104(2): 320-44.
[http://dx.doi.org/10.1590/S0074-02762009000200029] [PMID: 19430661]

[152]   Phan L, Kasza K, Jalbrzikowski J, *et al.* Toxoplasmosis Study Group. Longitudinal study of new eye lesions in treated congenital toxoplasmosis. Ophthalmology 2008; 115(3): 553-559.e8.

[153]   Koppe JG, Loewer-Sieger DH, de Roever-Bonnet H. Results of 20-year follow-up of congenital toxoplasmosis. Lancet 1986; 1(8475): 254-6.
[http://dx.doi.org/10.1016/S0140-6736(86)90785-3] [PMID: 2868264]

[154]   Phan L, Kasza K, Jalbrzikowski J, *et al.* Toxoplasmosis Study Group. Longitudinal study of new eye lesions in children with toxoplasmosis who were not treated during the first year of life. Am J Ophthalmol 2008; 146(3): 375-84.

[155]   Lebech M, Joynson DH, Seitz HM, *et al.* European Research Network on Congenital Toxoplasmosis. Classification system and case definitions of *Toxoplasma gondii* infection in immunocompetent pregnant women and their congenitally infected offspring. Eur J Clin Microbiol Infect Dis 1996; 15(10): 799-805.
[http://dx.doi.org/10.1007/BF01701522] [PMID: 8950557]

[156]   BRAZIL. Atenção à Saúde do Recém-Nascido. Guia para os Profissionais de Saúde. Intervenções Comuns, Icterícia e Infecções In: Saúde Md, editor. Brasília 2013. p. 167.

[157]   Diseases ACoI. Red Book, 29th Edition [2012 ]. Pickering LK, Baker CJ, Kimberlin DW, editors: American Academy of Pediatrics; 2012 2012-06-08 00:00:00. 1098 p.

[158]   Ferreira MU, Hiramoto RM, Aureliano DP, *et al.* A community-based survey of human toxoplasmosis in rural Amazonia: seroprevalence, seroconversion rate, and associated risk factors. Am J Trop Med Hyg 2009; 81(1): 171-6.

[159]   Vasconcelos-Santos DV, Machado Azevedo DO, Campos WR, *et al.* UFMG Congenital Toxoplasmosis Brazilian Group. Congenital toxoplasmosis in southeastern Brazil: results of early ophthalmologic examination of a large cohort of neonates. Ophthalmology 2009; 116(11): 2199-205.e1.

[160]   Dubey JP, Lago EG, Gennari SM, Su C, Jones JL. Toxoplasmosis in humans and animals in Brazil: high prevalence, high burden of disease, and epidemiology. Parasitology 2012; 139(11): 1375-424.
[http://dx.doi.org/10.1017/S0031182012000765] [PMID: 22776427]

[161]   Lago E, Carvalho R, Jungblut R, Silva V, Fiori R. Screening for *Toxoplasma gondii* antibodies in 2,513 consecutive parturient women and evaluation of newborn infants at risk for congenital toxoplasmosis. Sci Med 2009; 19(1): 27-34.

[162]   Melamed J, Dornelles F, Eckert GU. Alterações tomográficas cerebrais em crianças com lesões oculares por toxoplasmose congênita. J Pediatr 2001; 77: 475-480.162.

[163]   Resende L, Andrade G, Azevedo M, Perissimoto J, Vieira A. Congenital toxoplasmosis: auditory and language outcomes in early diagnosed and treated children. Sci Med 2010; 20(1): 13-9.

# CHAPTER 3

# Congenital Toxoplasmosis in Dogs

**Lucilene G. Camossi**[3,*], **Daniel F.F. Cardia**[3], **Celso T.N. Suzuki**[1], **Jancarlo F. Gomes**[1,2] and **Katia D.S. Bresciani**[3]

[1] *UNICAMP, Universidade Estadual de Campinas, Instituto de Computação, Campinas, São Paulo, Brazil*

[2] *UNICAMP, Universidade Estadual de Campinas, Faculdade de Ciências Médicas, Campinas, São Paulo, Brazil*

[3] *Universidade Estadual Paulista (Unesp) Faculdade de Medicina Veterinária de Araçatuba, Araçatuba, São Paulo, Brazil. Research ID E-7126-2012*

**Abstract:** *Toxoplasma gondii* is an apicomplexan protozoan parasite that infects a broad range of hosts, including dogs. Due to the high rate of dogs naturally infected with *T. gondii* and its correlation with immunosuppressive diseases, attention should be paid to the occurrence of this parasite in canine population, especially puppies, which are considered of high risk for developing the disease. Toxoplasmosis in puppies is particularly important, because the effects of the disease may have consequences on animals' lives, and they may have immeasurable value, being considered as family members. The main objective of this chapter will be to discuss important aspects involving congenital toxoplasmosis in this animal species.

**Keywords:** Clinical signs, Control, Dogs, Infection, Neurological alterations, Newborn, Opportunistic disease, Pathogeny, Pregnancy, Prevention, Puppies, PCR, Reproductive abnormalities, Serology, Treatment, Toxoplasmosis.

## INTRODUCTION

*Toxoplasma gondii* is a protozoan parasite that causes coccidiosis in domestic and wild felids [1, 2]. It is able to infect almost any warm-blooded animal [3], and is recognized to cause disease of high impact in public health and veterinary medicine, including livestock, wild and pet animals [4].

Serological studies in dogs have indicated that toxoplasmosis is widely distributed in canine population [4]. Although the clinical manifestation of toxoplasmosis is less common, it is recognized as an opportunistic disease in dogs related to immu-

* **Corresponding author Lucilene G. Camossi:** Faculdade de Medicina Veterinária de Araçatuba, Universidade Estadual Paulista "Júlio de Mesquita Filho", UNESP, Araçatuba, São Paulo, Brazil; Tel/Fax: +55 18 3636 1400; E-mail: lucilenecamossi@gmail.com

**Katia Denise Saraiva Bresciani & Alvimar José da Costa (Eds.)**

nosuppressive conditions [5], such as concomitant infections by *Leishmania* (*Leishmania*) *infantum chagasi* [6], Canine Distemper virus [5], and *Erlichia* spp [7]. The periparturient period has been associated with physiological immunosuppression in female dogs due to impaired cell-mediated and humoral immunity [8, 9] and its influence on opportunist infections. One of the major consequences of pregnant dogs becoming infected by *T. gondii* is the vertical transmission to fetuses.

Clinical manifestations of toxoplasmosis in dogs, when present, include mainly involvement of organs such as brain, lungs, liver and muscle [7]. Neurologic, respiratory, hepatic and muscular abnormalities can be seen, depending on the localization of the injury caused by the parasite, usually associated with focal necrosis lesions. The most severe disease occurs in pups [10] associated with congenital acquired toxoplasmosis. Although toxoplasmosis infection in the female dog may cause placentitis and eventually lead to abortion [7], more commonly it will damage the fetus, affecting the development of puppies.

## CONGENITAL TRANSMISSION

The prevalence of congenital toxoplasmosis in dogs is thought to be less common than in other animal species, such as sheep and goats [7]. Under experimental conditions the congenital transmission was demonstrated, when female dogs were infected with oocysts during pregnancy and *T. gondii* parasites were isolated from homogenized tissue of puppies and one female dog aborted [11].

Female dogs naturally infected with *T. gondii* were experimentally reinfected during pregnancy period with tachyzoites and oocysts. This study demonstrated that all reinfected female canines miscarried or presented fetal death [12]. It was shown that the repeated transmission of *T. gondii* may occur in subsequent pregnancies, even after the development of natural immunity after the primary infection.

The first description of a natural congenital transmission of *T. gondii* was described by Al-Qassab *et al.* [13]. In this study, it was found that all puppies from the litter contained *T. gondii* DNA in the brain tissue. Western blotting using anti-IgG and IgM showed that the female dog was probably infected during the pregnancy period, and genotyping confirmed the Type-II strain. It is recognized that the genotype of the strain of *T. gondii* may influence the clinical severity [14].

## PATOGENY AND CLINICAL SIGNS

Severity of congenital infection in female dogs varies with the stage of pregnancy they are infected. Obstetric signs include fetal death, resorption, abortion and premature parturition [15]. Healthy newborns and stillbirths can be observed in the same litter [12]. Severe and generalized toxoplasmosis characterized by fever, dyspnea, tonsillitis, diarrhea and vomiting is most commonly observed in puppies under one year of age. Hepatic involvement with extensive areas of necrosis can result in icterus [7].

Systemic signs in female dogs such as lymphadenopathy, digestive and respiratory disorders are observed, whereas pulmonary lesions represent the most common abnormality found in canine toxoplasmosis, mainly chronic pneumonia and diffuse bronchopneumonia [12]. Uterine disorders such as endometritis and placentitis have also been described [7, 12]. Severe clinical toxoplasmosis is seen in older dogs, and results in neurological deficit and muscular abnormalities. Neurological symptoms depend on the area of injury caused by the parasite and can include tremors, ataxia, paresis and paralysis. Muscular involvement may result in abnormal gait, staggering gait, muscle wasting, stiffness, paraparesis and tetraparesis [7].

## DIAGNOSIS

Suspicion of toxoplasmosis should be raised when neurologic, respiratory, digestive, muscular and reproductive abnormalities are detected. The diagnosis often depends on laboratory tests, due to toxoplasmosis in dogs mimicking the symptoms of many infectious diseases [16]. Furthermore, diagnosis of fetal infection is essential for the initiation of treatment, to minimize complications for extrauterine life.

IFAT and MAT are two serological tests of proven accuracy to detect anti-*T. gondii* antibodies in canine sera. The laboratory diagnosis of toxoplasmosis requires demonstration of high titers of specific antibodies and increasing levels in two serum samples taken two to four weeks apart [17].

The detection of parasite DNA in body tissue or fluids, as amniotic fluid, blood and placenta, may be performed by polymerase chain reaction (PCR).

Serological tests to detect anti-*T. gondii* antibodies when used in association with molecular methods may be more beneficial for accurate diagnosis of congenital toxoplasmosis [18].

## PREVENTION AND CONTROL

Prevalence of canine toxoplasmosis has been higher in countries where pets are usually fed with raw meat products [7]. Thus, the main control measure is preventing ingestion of raw meat, and pregnant female dogs should preferably be fed with commercially processed food. If the dog is fed with homemade food, the fresh meat should be cooked at a temperature of at least 60 °C to 100 °C for 10 minutes. Freezing meat at −10 °C for three days or at −20 °C for two days prior to feeding is sufficient to kill tissue cysts of *T. gondii*. However, neither cooking in a microwave nor chilling at 5 °C for five days is sufficient to inactivate the parasite [19].

Female dogs should not be exposed to feline feces. Dogs should be kept away from the litter box to prevent ingestion of oocysts [20], either through accidental ingestion or coprophagia behaviour. Also, special attention should be given to the water supplied to animals, which must be clean or treated [21].

Street access may favor hunting chances, inherent to the behavior of a carnivorous animal. Therefore, pregnant dogs should be monitored in outdoor activities or be restricted to prevent hunting and ingestion of potential intermediate hosts, for example, rodents and birds [7, 22].

## TREATMENT

The pharmaceutical options commonly used to treat toxoplasmosis are protozoastatic, which suppress only the tachyzoite stage. They are not effective in eliminating the cyst stage of *T. gondii* from the host, and thus they do not prevent recurrence of the disease [23].

Treatment protocols with available drugs for canine toxoplasmosis include clindamycin, trimethoprim, and sulfa combinations, such as sulfadimidine used together with pyrimethamine or a combination of sulfadimidine and trimethoprim [24]. Azithromycin and ponazuril are also effective to treat the infection. Clindamycin has been successfully used to treat fever, myositis, uveitis, and neuropathies in animals, even though gastrointestinal irritation can occur in some treated animals [25].

## CONCLUDING REMARKS

Toxoplasmosis infection in pregnant dogs may produce spontaneous abortion, but more commonly causes developmental problems that will impact the life of puppies, especially under one year of age. *T. gondii* spreads systematically and affects various organs, which can result in a wide range of clinical signs. Neurological, respiratory, digestive, muscular and reproductive abnormalities should raise the suspicion of clinical toxoplasmosis. Laboratory diagnosis of toxoplasmosis is of primary importance to determine the treatment. The combination of serology and PCR are efficient and accurate tools to confirm the diagnosis.

## CONSENT FOR PUBLICATION

Not applicable.

## CONFLICT OF INTEREST

The authors declare no conflict of interest, financial or otherwise.

## ACKNOWLEDGEMENTS

Declared none.

## REFERENCES

[1]     Dubey JP. History of the discovery of the life cycle of *Toxoplasma gondii.* Int J Parasitol 2009; 39(8): 877-82.
        [http://dx.doi.org/10.1016/j.ijpara.2009.01.005] [PMID: 19630138]

[2]     Dubey JP, Lindsay DS, Lappin MR. Toxoplasmosis and other intestinal coccidial infections in cats and dogs. Vet Clin North Am Small Anim Pract 2009; 39(6): 1009-1034, v.
        [http://dx.doi.org/10.1016/j.cvsm.2009.08.001] [PMID: 19932360]

[3]     Boothroyd JC. Expansion of host range as a driving force in the evolution of *Toxoplasma.* Mem Inst Oswaldo Cruz 2009; 104(2): 179-84.
        [http://dx.doi.org/10.1590/S0074-02762009000200009] [PMID: 19430641]

[4]     Dubey JP. Toxoplasmosis of Animals and Humans. 2nd ed., Boca Raton: CRC Press Taylor & Francis Group 2010.

[5]     Moretti Ld, Da Silva AV, Ribeiro MG, Paes AC, Langoni H. *Toxoplasma gondii* genotyping in a dog co-infected with distemper virus and ehrlichiosis rickettsia. Rev Inst Med Trop São Paulo 2006; 48(6): 359-63.
        [http://dx.doi.org/10.1590/S0036-46652006000600012] [PMID: 17221136]

[6]     Sakamoto KP, de Melo GD, Machado GF. T and B lymphocytes in the brains of dogs with concomitant seropositivity to three pathogenic protozoans: *Leishmania chagasi*, *Toxoplasma gondii* and *Neospora caninum*. BMC Res Notes 2013; 6: 226.
        [http://dx.doi.org/10.1186/1756-0500-6-226] [PMID: 23758819]

[7]     Dubey JP, Lappin MR. Toxoplasmosis and neosporosis.Greene CE Infectious diseases of the dog and cat. Saint Louis: Saunders Elsevier 2006; pp. 754-75.

[8]     Lloyd S, Amerasinghe H, Soulsby JL. Periparturient immunosuppression in the bitch and its influence on infection with *Toxocara canis*. J Small Anim Pract 1983; 24(4): 237-47.
        [http://dx.doi.org/10.1111/j.1748-5827.1983.tb00437.x]

[9]     Panciera DL, Troy GC, Purswell BJ. Blastomycosis in a postpartum dog. Med Mycol Case Rep 2014; 6: 29-30.
        [http://dx.doi.org/10.1016/j.mmcr.2014.09.002] [PMID: 25379395]

[10]    Dubey JP, Jones JL. *Toxoplasma gondii* infection in humans and animals in the United States. Int J Parasitol 2008; 38(11): 1257-78.
        [http://dx.doi.org/10.1016/j.ijpara.2008.03.007] [PMID: 18508057]

[11]    Bresciani KD, Costa AJ, Toniollo GH, *et al.* Experimental toxoplasmosis in pregnant bitches. Vet Parasitol 1999; 86(2): 143-5.

[http://dx.doi.org/10.1016/S0304-4017(99)00136-3] [PMID: 10496698]

[12]   Bresciani KD, Costa AJ, Toniollo GH, *et al.* Transplacental transmission of *Toxoplasma gondii* in reinfected pregnant female canines. Parasitol Res 2009; 104(5): 1213-7.
[http://dx.doi.org/10.1007/s00436-008-1317-5] [PMID: 19137327]

[13]   Al-Qassab S, Reichel MP, Su C, *et al.* Isolation of *Toxoplasma gondii* from the brain of a dog in Australia and its biological and molecular characterization. Vet Parasitol 2009; 164(2-4): 335-9.
[http://dx.doi.org/10.1016/j.vetpar.2009.05.019] [PMID: 19556061]

[14]   Robert-Gangneux F, Dardé ML. Epidemiology of and diagnostic strategies for toxoplasmosis. Clin Microbiol Rev 2012; 25(2): 264-96.
[http://dx.doi.org/10.1128/CMR.05013-11] [PMID: 22491772]

[15]   Bresciani KD, Toniollo GH, Costa AJ, Sabatini GA, Moraes FR. Clinical, parasitological and obstetric observations in pregnant bitches with experimental toxoplasmosis. Cienc Rural 2001; 31(6): 1039-43.
[http://dx.doi.org/10.1590/S0103-84782001000600020]

[16]   Dubey JP. Toxoplasmosis in dogs. Canine Pract 1985; 12(6): 7-28.

[17]   Dubey JP. Toxoplasmosis. Vet Clin North Am Small Anim Pract 1987; 17(6): 1389-404.
[http://dx.doi.org/10.1016/S0195-5616(87)50008-0] [PMID: 3328395]

[18]   Stiles J, Prade R, Greene C. Detection of *Toxoplasma gondii* in feline and canine biological samples by use of the polymerase chain reaction. Am J Vet Res 1996; 57(3): 264-7.
[PMID: 8669752]

[19]   El-Nawawi FA, Tawfik MA, Shaapan RM. Methods for inactivation of *Toxoplasma gondii* cysts in meat and tissues of experimentally infected sheep. Foodborne Pathog Dis 2008; 5(5): 687-90.
[http://dx.doi.org/10.1089/fpd.2007.0060] [PMID: 18681796]

[20]   Lopez A, Dietz VJ, Wilson M, Navin TR, Jones JL. Preventing congenital toxoplasmosis.Centers for Disease Control and Prevention CDC Recommendations Regarding Selected Conditions Affecting Women's Health. Atlanta: Centers for Disease Control and Prevention 2000; pp. 59-68.

[21]   Jones JL, Dubey JP. Foodborne toxoplasmosis. Clin Infect Dis 2012; 55(6): 845-51.
[http://dx.doi.org/10.1093/cid/cis508] [PMID: 22618566]

[22]   Esch KJ, Petersen CA. Transmission and epidemiology of zoonotic protozoal diseases of companion animals. Clin Microbiol Rev 2013; 26(1): 58-85.
[http://dx.doi.org/10.1128/CMR.00067-12] [PMID: 23297259]

[23]   Swinger RL, Schmidt KA Jr, Dubielzig RR. Keratoconjunctivitis associated with *Toxoplasma gondii* in a dog. Vet Ophthalmol 2009; 12(1): 56-60.
[http://dx.doi.org/10.1111/j.1463-5224.2009.00675.x] [PMID: 19152600]

[24]   Dubey JP, Lappin MR. Toxoplasmosis and neosporosis. Infectious diseases of the dog and cat. Saint Louis: Saunders Elsevier 2012; pp. 806-27.

[25]   Greene CE, Cook JR Jr, Mahaffey EA. Clindamycin for treatment of *Toxoplasma* polymyositis in a dog. J Am Vet Med Assoc 1985; 187(6): 631-4.
[PMID: 4086374]

# CHAPTER 4

# Congenital Toxoplasmosis in Cats

**André L. B. Galvão[1,*], Victor J. V. Rosseto[1], Breno C. Cruz[2], Weslen F. P. Teixeira[3], Alvimar J. da Costa[2] and Katia D. S. Bresciani[2,3]**

*[1] UNIRP, Centro Universitário de Rio Preto, Faculdade de Medicina Veterinária, São José do Rio Preto, São Paulo, Brazil*

*[2] Universidade Estadual Paulista (Unesp) Faculdade de Ciências Agrárias e Veterinárias de Jaboticabal, CPPAR, Centro de Pesquisas em Saúde Animal, Jaboticabal, SP, Brazil*

*[3] Universidade Estadual Paulista (Unesp), Faculdade de Medicina Veterinária de Araçatuba, Araçatuba, São Paulo, Brazil*

**Abstract:** *Toxoplasma gondii* is a protozoan which commonly infects cats, dogs and humans, causing toxoplasmosis. This disease, of great importance in public health, is acquired by consumption of meat and by-products containing cysts, ingestion of food and/or water contaminated with oocysts, as well as through the placenta. Congenital *Toxoplasma* infections are reported in many species, being relevant in both medicine and veterinary medicine. In cats, congenital toxoplasmosis is associated with the occurrence of injuries in the liver, lungs, central nervous system and eyes, observed when hosts are infected in the middle to the last thirds of pregnancy. Ocular form can occur in young cats, infected through placenta, with no other clinical signs. The objective of this chapter is to describe the main manifestations of congenital toxoplasmosis in cats.

**Keywords:** Antibodies, Blindness, Chorioretinitis, Clinical signs, Diagnosis, Epidemiology, Feline, Immunity, Miscarriages, Newborn, Pathology, Pregnancy, Prevention, Prognosis, Queen, Stillbirths, Transmission, Treatment, Uveitis.

## INTRODUCTION

Domestic cats, as well as other felines, may be intermediate or definitive hosts of *Toxoplasma gondii*. Once oocysts are excreted, they will become infective in the environment, under optimal conditions such as temperature and humidity [1, 2].

---

*\* Corresponding author André L. B. Galvão: UNESP, Universidade Estadual Paulista Julio de Mesquita Filho, Faculdade de Ciências Agrárias e Veterinárias de Jaboticabal, Jaboticabal, SP, Brazil;
E-mail: andrelgalvao@hotmail.com

**Katia Denise Saraiva Bresciani & Alvimar José da Costa (Eds.)**

Most *T. gondii* isolates are grouped into three major genotypes classified as types I, II and III. The type I isolate is normally associated to ocular disease and congenital infection in humans. On the other hand, types II and III are commonly observed in infected [2] animals.

An important zoonotic disease, of particular interest in public health, toxoplasmosis, can be transmitted by the intake of infected meat containing tissue cysts with bradyzoites, or through water and raw food contaminated with infective oocysts [2]. The congenital form of toxoplasmosis has great importance in human and veterinary medicine, as it is related to the occurrence of premature births or stillbirths, and to the development of severe lesions involving the central nervous system [3]. Infections with *T. gondii* in cats are usually asymptomatic at least 17 species of wild felines have been reported to shed oocysts of *T. gondii*, European and African wild cats, Pallas cat, bobcat, leopard cat, Amur leopard cat, iriomote cat, ocelot, Geoffroy's cat, Pampas cat, jaguarundi, cougar, leopard, jaguar, tiger, lion and cheetah, and there is serological evidence of *T. gondii* infection in servals [4, 5]. The cats deserve special attention regarding their role in epidemiology and dissemination of toxoplasmosis, however, in feline medicine the congenital form of toxoplasmosis is little approached, constituting the objective of this study.

## EPIDEMIOLOGY

The congenital form of toxoplasmosis is characterized by vertical transmission of *T. gondii* to fetuses through the placenta [4, 5]. Sixteen pregnant queens were inoculated orally with the tissue cysts of *T. gondii,* and fetal membranes and offspring were examined for *T. gondii.* They were isolated from the tissues of seven of 33 fetuses [5]. The maternal immunity of domestic cats did not protect the kittens against infection with *T. gondii* and that maternal immunity might not have prevented transplacental transmission of the parasite [6].

*T. gondii* is transmitted through 3 primary routes in cats: by ingestion of tissue cysts, by contamination through oocysts from infected cat feces, or through congenital infection. Other minor modes of transmission include lactational and transfusion of body fluids [2, 5 - 7].

Tachyzoites, which break the placental barrier, are acquired by mothers through traditional ways of *Toxoplasma* infection. Recently, it is believed that the parasite can infect females during sex, through exposure to seminal fluids of infected males [7, 8]. Sexual transmission in domestic cats does not appear to be an important route of infection by *T. gondii,* and the presence of this coccidium was not detected in semen, testicle and epididymis tissues of cats experimentally infected by this coccidium, in none of the experiments [9].

Congenital toxoplasmosis has been observed in several animal species, including humans and domestic cats. Its occurrence is dependent on the type of isolate, challenge levels and the stage of fetal development during infection [5].

In cats, congenital form of toxoplasmosis is a constant target of studies. However, serological monitoring of queens is not a reality during pregnancy, and sometimes kittens may present antibodies titers that cannot be detected. Also, the isolation of parasite in placenta is usually not possible due to the feline's habit of eating it soon after birth [4, 10].

Unlike what happens in humans, clinical manifestations of congenital toxoplasmosis in felines are usually described when the pregnant female is infected in the final third of gestation [6, 10].

## PATHOGENESIS AND CLINICAL SIGNS

Clinical manifestations of congenital toxoplasmosis are also dependent on the type of isolate, challenge levels, stage of fetal development and the infectious stage of the parasite [5, 10].

The presence of inflammatory infiltrate, with predominance of macrophages and neutrophils, is described in injuries involving nervous tissues of cats infected through the congenital route. These injured areas are usually discrete and multifocal, more often affecting perivascular spaces of the brain and spinal cord, followed by the cerebellum. Tissue cysts and areas of necrosis are rare and, generally, nodular gliosis forms secondary to vasculitis, since tachyzoites replicate in capillary endothelium [4].

In one study, 21 newborn cats, as pregnant queens, were infected during middle and late pregnancy, and were diagnosed at autopsy with macroscopic injuries in the livers and lungs of 90% and 48%, respectively, in the animals. In histopathological evaluation, the inflammatory infiltrates, predominantly composed of macrophages and neutrophils, with necrosis areas, were observed in all the evaluated animals [4]. The most commonly affected organs were the liver, lungs, central nervous system and eyes [2].

Congenitally infected cats usually present lethargy, depression, hypothermia, ascites, encephalitis, pneumonia and uveitis. In severe cases, sudden death occurs within a few days of life [2, 4]. On the other hand, enteritis, caused by injuries to intestinal epithelium, and lymphadenopathy are not verified. These findings are normally observed in cats infected in the postnatal period, mainly orally [4].

Uveitis occurs due to intraocular migration and replication of intracellular tachyzoites, which damage the uveal tract, retina and optic nerve, due to disruption of cellular plasma membranes and deposition of immunocomplexes [4, 5]. Consequently, an exudative inflammatory process takes place characterized by uveitis and, in more severe cases, retinal detachment [2].

This pathway is confirmed by studies, which conducted parasite's DNA by means of PCR, on the aqueous humor from naturally or experimentally infected cats [11]. However, although there was an intraocular migration of *T. gondii*, hosts not always expressed signs of uveitis, and the reason why some cats developed ocular form, while others did not, remained uncertain [9].

Among ocular manifestations present in uveitis induced by toxoplasmosis, the following signs can be observed: formation of "flare" in aqueous humor, keratic precipitates and lens shift. In severe cases, with the progression of inflammation, glaucoma caused by iridocorneal drainage angle obstruction is also present [2]. Obstruction caused by deposition of precipitated protein results in preventing the flow of produced aqueous humor, which accumulates, leading to an increase in intraocular pressure and distension of the eye coats [12].

An increase in intraocular pressure can irreversibly injure the retina and nervous tissues, with the occurrence of blindness. Thus, cats with glaucoma secondary to toxoplasmosis may also present buftalmia, congestion of episcleral vessels, reduction of tear production due to eye inflammation, formation of corneal striae and ulcerative keratitis by decreased tear production and ocular surface exposure, with unresponsive mydriasis to the pupillary reflex [12].

Ocular form of the disease can occur without manifestation of other clinical signs in young cats infected transplacentally, and is mainly dependent on the type of isolate, with some types having higher tropism for ocular tissue when compared to others [5, 10].

In fact, in a study evaluating frequency and severity of eye injuries in newborn cats from females experimentally infected during pregnancy, about 72% of the animals had consistent chorioretinitis lesions, while only 14% showed other clinical changes in physical exams [10]. Amongst cats with ocular lesions, more severe lesions were observed in animals infected by the Mozart type, while those affected by ME-49 and Meggie serotypes had focal and smaller lesions, confined to the tapetal zone [10].

Manifestation and severity of clinical disease also depend on the gestational period in which infection occurs [10]. Therefore, when pregnant female cats are infected in the final third of pregnancy, usually there are systemic clinical manifestations [6, 10]. When infected in the first third of pregnancy, it is common to observe the occurrence of abortion and stillbirths [13].

## DIAGNOSIS

After *T. gondii* infection, humoral immune response is observed with the production of antibodies detectable by IFAT, IHA, MAT and ELISA. Additionally, the presence of tachyzoites can be detected by cytology examination of body fluids such as blood, cerebrospinal fluid, bronchoalveolar lavage fluid and ascites and pleural effusion [2]. Infective forms of the parasite can still be observed through histopathological and immunohistochemical examinations; both are usually performed during necropsy [4]. There are, however, no clinic or pathological changes in pathognomonic of congenital toxoplasmosis, and the definitive diagnosis depends on the identification of the parasite and positive serodiagnosis [14]. Detection of nucleic acid sequences using techniques for detecting protozoa in clinical research projects is based on polymerase chain reaction, which can be used to verify the presence of *T. gondii* in biologic specimens [2]. Polymerase chain reaction was more sensitive than the mouse inoculation bioassay for detecting infection in the blood of experimentally infected cats [2]. Identification of *T. gondii* specific IgM antibody and organism by polymerase chain reaction in cerebrospinal fluid or aqueous humor of symptomatic animals suggests toxoplasmosis [2].

## TREATMENT

Treatment of infected cats includes clindamycin administration by oral or parenteral routes, with alleviation of clinical signs in 24 to 48 hours after beginning the treatment. Ocular changes, however, show improvement of their clinical state only after one week of treatment [2].

Clindamycin is also indicated for treatment of infected pregnant cats, as it crosses the placenta barrier and is excreted in milk, resulting in shorter periods of oocyst shedding in feces [15, 16]. Recommended dosages of clindamycin for cats range from 5.5 to 11 mg/kg, orally, intramuscular or intravenous every 12 hours, or from 25 to 50 mg/kg orally every 24 hours. The minimum duration of treatment is two to three weeks [15]. High doses can result in irritation of digestive tract, with clinical manifestations such as anorexia, vomit and diarrhea [2]. Additionally, combinations of trimethoprim with sulfamethoxazole, or other pyrimethamine with sulfonamides, have also been effective in treating congenital toxoplasmosis [2, 17], especially for ocular forms of this disease in humans [2].

The recommended dose of trimethoprim with sulfamethoxazole associations for cats is 30 mg/kg orally every 12 hours, and the minimum treatment time is 21 days [15]. High doses for prolonged periods may result in keratoconjunctivitis sicca, mental depression and renal failure due to bone marrow suppression, anemia, leukopenia and thrombocytopenia. Therefore, hematological monitoring by serum biochemical profile is recommended [2, 15]. In addition, high doses have teratogenic effects and should not be given to infected female cats during pregnancy [15].

However, there are no reports of cats treated for congenital toxoplasmosis with these mentioned drugs, and in most experimental studies, the objective is either the histopathological evaluation of animals that are euthanized, or analysis of the natural course of the disease [4, 9].

## PROGNOSIS

After systemic clinical manifestations, prognosis of congenital toxoplasmosis, when adequate treatment is not instituted, is reserved to poor, depending on severity of injuries, evolving to death within eight days after birth [6]. Likewise, the resolution of ocular form depends on extension and severity of lesions, and tends to occur in two to four weeks, eventually taking up to nine weeks after the onset of signs [10]. Sequelae may, however, occur in large inflammation areas due to discoloration or hyperreflexia of tapetal zone [10].

## PREVENTION

The prevention of congenital toxoplasmosis is very important and should be done in humans, with monthly serological monitoring, or at least every three months, of the mother entering the first trimester of pregnancy, thereby preventing vertical transmission and risks of sequelae to the fetus [1]. In veterinary medicine, preventing toxoplasmosis in dogs and cats involves measures intended to reduce the incidence of feline infections and subsequent shedding of oocysts to the environment. Kittens raised outdoors usually become infected shortly after they are weaned and begin to hunt. Cats should preferably be fed only dry or canned, or commercially processed cat food [2]. It is also important to minimize opportunities for coprophagia by cats, along with the control of insects and rodents in the environment [2].

## CONSENT FOR PUBLICATION

Not applicable.

## CONFLICT OF INTEREST

The authors declare no conflict of interest, financial or otherwise.

# ACKNOWLEDGEMENTS

Declared none.

# REFERENCES

[1]    Robert-Gangneux F. It is not only the cat that did it: how to prevent and treat congenital toxoplasmosis. J Infect 2014; 68 (Suppl. 1): S125-33.
[http://dx.doi.org/10.1016/j.jinf.2013.09.023] [PMID: 24119928]

[2]    Dubey JP, Lappin MR. Toxoplasmosis and neosporosis. Infectious diseases of the dog and cat. St. Louis: Elsevier 2006; p. 754.

[3]    Doudou Y, Renaud P, Coralie L, *et al.* Toxoplasmosis among pregnant women: high seroprevalence and risk factors in Kinshasa, Democratic Republic of Congo. Asian Pac J Trop Biomed 2014; 4(1): 69-74.
[http://dx.doi.org/10.1016/S2221-1691(14)60211-2] [PMID: 24144134]

[4]    Dubey JP, Mattix ME, Lipscomb TP. Lesions of neonatally induced toxoplasmosis in cats. Vet Pathol 1996; 33(3): 290-5.
[http://dx.doi.org/10.1177/030098589603300305] [PMID: 8740702]

[5]    Dubey JP, Lappin MR, Thulliez P. Diagnosis of induced toxoplasmosis in neonatal cats. J Am Vet Med Assoc 1995; 207(2): 179-85.
[PMID: 7601711]

[6]    Bresciani KD, Galvão AL, Vasconcelllos AL, *et al.* Neonatal Toxoplasmosis in Dogs and Kittens.Recent Advances in Toxoplasmosis Research. Nova Science Publishers 2013; p. 103.

[7]    Flegr J, Klapilová K, Kaňková S. Toxoplasmosis can be a sexually transmitted infection with serious clinical consequences. Not all routes of infection are created equal. Med Hypotheses 2014; 83(3): 286-9.
[http://dx.doi.org/10.1016/j.mehy.2014.05.019] [PMID: 24986706]

[8]    Bayat PD, Eslamirad Z, Shojaee S. Toxoplasmosis: experimental vaginal infections in NMRI mice and its effect on uterin, placenta and fetus tissues. Iran Red Crescent Med J 2013; 15(7): 595-9.
[http://dx.doi.org/10.5812/ircmj.11427] [PMID: 24396580]

[9]    Teixeira WF, Tozato ME, Pierucci JC, *et al.* Investigation of *Toxoplasma gondii* in semen, testicle and epididymis tissues of primo-infected cats (Felis catus). Vet Parasitol 2017; 238(238): 90-3.
[http://dx.doi.org/10.1016/j.vetpar.2017.04.003] [PMID: 28404209]

[10]   Powell CC, Lappin MR. Clinical ocular toxoplasmosis in neonatal kittens. Vet Ophthalmol 2001; 4(2): 87-92.
[http://dx.doi.org/10.1046/j.1463-5224.2001.00180.x] [PMID: 11422988]

[11]   Burney DP, Chavkin MJ, Dow SW, Potter TA, Lappin MR. Polymerase chain reaction for the detection of *Toxoplasma gondii* within aqueous humor of experimentally-inoculated cats. Vet Parasitol 1998; 79(3): 181-6.
[http://dx.doi.org/10.1016/S0304-4017(98)00172-1] [PMID: 9823058]

[12]   Brooks DE. Glaucoma. Oftalmologia clínica em animais de companhia. São Paulo: Med Vet 2008; p. 195.

[13]   Sakamoto CA, da Costa AJ, Gennari SM, *et al.* Experimental infection of pregnant queens with two major Brazilian clonal lineages of *Toxoplasma gondii.* Parasitol Res 2009; 105(5): 1311-6.
[http://dx.doi.org/10.1007/s00436-009-1558-y] [PMID: 19629528]

[14]   Carvalho AC, Pacheco MR, Baraldi-Artoni SM, Girardi AM. Toxoplasmosis: morphological and morphometric evaluation of spinal cord neurons from nonsymptomatic seropositive dogs. Cienc Anim Bras 2015; 16: 225-34.

[http://dx.doi.org/10.1590/1089-6891v16i218991]

[15]    Andrade SF, Giuffrida R, Ribeiro MG. Quimioterápicos antimicrobianos e antibióticos. Manual de Terapêutica Veterinária. São Paulo: Roca 2002; p. 13.

[16]    Swinger RL, Schmidt KA Jr, Dubielzig RR. Keratoconjunctivitis associated with *Toxoplasma gondii* in a dog. Vet Ophthalmol 2009; 12(1): 56-60.
         [http://dx.doi.org/10.1111/j.1463-5224.2009.00675.x] [PMID: 19152600]

[17]    Papich MG. Manual Saunders: Terapêutico Veterinário. 2nd ed., São Paulo: MedVet 2009.

# CHAPTER 5

# Congenital Toxoplasmosis in Ewes

**Thaís Rabelo dos Santos**[1,*], **Maerle Oliveira Maia**[2], **Alvimar José da Costa**[3] and **Katia Denise Saraiva Bresciani**[4]

*[1] UFVJM, Universidade Federal dos Vales do Jequitinhonha e Mucuri, Instituto de Ciências Agrárias, Unaí, Minas Gerais, Brasil*

*[2] UFMT, Universidade Federal do Mato Grosso, Faculdade de Medicina Veterinária, Cuiabá, Mato Grosso, Brasil*

*[3] Universidade Estadual Paulista (Unesp), Faculdade de Ciências Agrárias e Veterinárias de Jaboticabal, CPPAR, Centro de Pesquisas em Sanidade Animal, Jaboticabal, São Paulo, Brasil*

*[4] Universidade Estadual Paulista (Unesp), Faculdade de Medicina Veterinária de Araçatuba, Araçatuba, São Paulo, Brasil*

**Abstract:** *T. gondii* is prevalent in most areas of the world and is of veterinary and medical importance, because it may cause abortion or congenital disease in its intermediate hosts. In sheep, *T. gondii* is an important cause of abortion, which can result in considerable economic losses. Herbivores acquire infection mainly by the ingestion of oocysts in water or contaminated food. Seroprevalence of *T. gondii* in sheep have been reported extensively in different countries and the positive rates ranged from 3% to 95%. The diagnosis of toxoplasmosis can be made by means of indirect methods such as serological evaluation to detect specific antibodies. The hypothesis that primary infection protects against reinfection is the basis for many farmers not to discard sheep with a history of abortion. However, recent studies have suggested that sheep persistently infected with *T. gondii* may transmit the infection congenitally more frequently than expected. Ewes persistently infected with c transmitted the infection congenitally, possibly due to an acute relapse process. This result shows that the immunity acquired in the primary infection did not protect the ewes against future *T. gondii* reinfections. The experimental *T. gondii* reinfection triggered severe reproductive alterations (locomotive changes, malformations, stillbirths and disability) in Santa Inês ewes primarily infected at different pregnancy stages. Therefore, congenital *T. gondii* infection was common when ewes were chronically infected prior to pregnancy, with or without reinfection during at various stages of gestation.

**Keywords:** Congenital Toxoplasmosis, Ewes, Pregnancy, *Toxoplasma gondii*.

---

* **Corresponding author Thaís Rabelo dos Santos:** UFVJM, Universidade Federal dos Vales do Jequitinhonha e Mucuri, Instituto de Ciências Agrárias, Unaí, Minas Gerais, Brasil; Tel/Fax: 055 43 33714766; E-mail: rabelo.vet@hotmail.com

# INTRODUCTION

The tissue cyst-forming coccidium *Toxoplasma gondii* is one of the more polyxenous parasites known to date. It has a facultatively heteroxenous life cycle and can probably infect all warm-blooded animals (mammals and birds) and humans. *T. gondii* is prevalent in most areas of the world and is of veterinary and medical importance, because it may cause abortion or congenital disease in its intermediate hosts. Because of its great importance as a causative agent of a zoonosis *T. gondii* has been studied most intensively among the coccidia [1].

The sheep toxoplasmosis was first described by [2], in the United States. These authors reported this disease in a female with nervous symptoms, hyperthermia, muscular rigidity, among other clinical signs. The diagnosis was established after necropsy and histopathological examination of the brain and spinal cord of the animal.

In sheep, *T. gondii* is an important cause of abortion, which can result in considerable economic losses [3].

# EPIDEMIOLOGY

In small ruminants, toxoplasmosis is common [4], it is responsible for reproductive problems causing great economic losses in sheep flocks [5, 6], in which infection becomes the main cause of miscarriages, fetal malformations, premature animals and stillbirths.

Herbivores acquire infection mainly by the ingestion of oocysts in water or contaminated food. Carnivores and omnivores, including human beings, can additionally become infected by ingesting meat with cysts (bradyzoites) or even tachyzoites [7]

Seroprevalence of *T. gondii* in sheep have been reported extensively in different countries and the positive rates ranged from 3% to 95% [8]. In Brazil, infection rates for sheep range from 8% to 55% (Nishikawa *et al.*, 1984) a 55% (Langoni *et al.*, 1999). This variation in occurrence occurs due to the type of serological test used, the region and the age of the animals studied (Dubey, 1990). The high occurrence of toxoplasmosis in sheep may be related to the lower resistance of this species to the parasite and the conditions of exploitation of sheep that offer a greater risk of exposure and contact of these animals with oocysts eliminated by cats (Dubey & Hamir, 2002).

Consumption of undercooked or raw meat presents the transmission risk of the parasite and this might be considered as an important public health problem, mainly for high-risk groups such as the pregnant and the immunodeficient [9].

## DIAGNOSIS

The diagnosis of toxoplasmosis can be made by means of indirect methods such as serological evaluation to detect specific antibodies. The most used diagnostic tests in 35-year surveys for sheep were indirect immunofluorescent assay (IFA), direct agglutination test (DAT), IHA, MAT, latex agglutination test (LAT) and Elisa [10].

The IFA is the most used test for the diagnosis of toxoplasmosis, being used as a gold standard. Therefore, titers of 16 or greater were considered positive for *T. gondii* (Dubey e Beattie, 1988). Currently, positive titles are considered to be greater than or equal to 64 (Costa *et al.*, 1977; Souza, 2001). Uchôa *et al.* (1999) detected sensitivity of 83.87% and specificity of 79.16% for IFA.

In the acute phase of toxoplasmosis, immunoglobulin M (IgM) production first occurs, followed by production of immunoglobulin G (IgG The infection may also produce immunoglobulin A (IgA) if the transmission has been orally. IgA antibodies can be titrated 1 to 2 weeks after infection onset, peaking at 6 to 8 weeks, when they decline. Low titles may persist for more than 12 months. IgG antibody persists throughout life in most patients (Goldsmith, 1998).

According to Santos *et al.*, 2010 [11], IFA has proved more effective than immunohistochemistry to detect positive and negative results of toxoplasmosis. These authors suggest that the use of IFA in mouse bioassays can be recommended without the need for evaluation of brain cysts, which is extremely difficult and laborious.

## CONGENITAL TOXOPLASMOSIS

Infections acquired early in pregnancy (before 50 days), before the foetus develops the ability to produce antibodies, typically cause embryonic death and reabsorption [12]. If the ewe becomes infected with *T. gondii* in them middle of pregnancy (70–90 days), there is a considerable probability of miscarriage or stillbirth [13 - 15], while in late pregnancy (>110 days) ewes will give birth normally, although their offspring may be congenitally infected [7, 9, 14 - 16]. However, few studies have described the occurrence of newborn lambs that are healthy but infected with *T. gondii* in ewe populations [17].

In humans *T. gondii* infection generates strong immunity to reinfection, limiting future congenital transmission during the next pregnancies, and any subsequently generated children will not be infected (Frenkel, 1990). Experimental vaccine studies using attenuated "S48" strain from *T. gondii* were successful in limiting the severity of congenital diseases when sheep were challenged with oocysts (Buxton e Innes, 1995). However, despite the success of vaccination in limiting congenital disease and abortion, this does not necessarily block the transmission of the disease (Buxton e Innes, 1995). It has also been shown that an oral dose of infective oocysts inoculated prior to gestation was sufficient to produce an immune response and consequently neutralize the parasitic challenge (McColgan *et al.*, 1988).

The hypothesis that primary infection protects against reinfection is the basis for many farmers not to discard sheep with a history of abortion. However, recent studies have suggested that sheep persistently infected with *T. gondii* may transmit the infection congenitally more frequently than expected [3].

Recently, several articles were published by a group of researchers in England [17 - 20]. These authors proposed that transplacental transmissions repeated by *T. gondii* in sheep may be more common than previously believed.

Congenital transmission at high occurrence rates (61%) was found in commercial herds (placenta and fetal tissues) using Polymerase Chain Reaction (PCR). *T. gondii* was isolated in 94% of pregnancies that resulted in deaths and 42% of those who came to term [17].

Williams *et al.* (2005) [19] detected high levels of congenital transmission in Charollais ewes (50.5%) and in commercial herds, without breeding (69%) by PCR. However, it was not possible to verify if the congenital transmission occurred in the first infection or with the reactivation of the chronic infection during the gestation, however the authors suggest that due to the high levels of transmission there must have been reactivation of toxoplasmosis.

According to Morley *et al.* (2005) [18], one hypothesis is that the vertical transmission of *T. gondii* occurs from generation to generation after a primary infection, resulting in the maintenance of high levels of infection in some families, while in others it does not. This pattern is mimicked by the occurrence of abortion in the same families due to the strong correlation between infection and abortion. The belief that *T. gondii* can be transmitted to descendants of infected family strains over successive generations is controversial, but should not be ruled out.

According to Morley *et al.* (2007) [20] there is a high risk (55%) of producing a stillbirth after a previous abortion, probably associated with toxoplasmosis. It is also reported that one-third of the diagnosed sheep abortions are related to *T. gondii* infection. This work reports the need for further studies on the acquired immunity of *T. gondii* throughout life, as well as its transmission to offspring.

These studies confirm the congenital transmission, however, there is no detailed study on primoinfection, reactivation of chronic infection or reinfection during pregnancy. In addition, all these studies are based on DNA detection by PCR of the placenta and fetal tissues.

Rodger *et al.* (2006) [21] failed to detect congenital transmission in persistently infected sheep. Thirty-one sheep naturally seropositive for *T. gondii* and 15 seronegative ewes were mated and monitored during gestation. No evidence of toxoplasmosis was found in the histopathology or PCR of the placenta or tissues of lambs. Low titers for the parasite were found in three lambs, but it was not possible to establish whether these antibodies represent evidence of fetal infection.

Life-long immunity to *T. gondii* infections may not always be acquired following an initial infection and raises the question as to whether the mechanisms of *T. gondii* transmission prior to and during ovine pregnancies are fully understood [20].

Ewes persistently infected with *T. gondii* transmitted the infection congenitally, possibly due to an acute relapse process. This result shows that the immunity acquired in the primary infection did not protect the ewes against future *T. gondii* reinfections. The experimental *T. gondii* reinfection triggered severe reproductive alterations (locomotive changes, malformations, stillbirths and disability) in Santa Inês ewes primarily infected at different pregnancy stages. Therefore, congenital *T. gondii* infection was common when ewes were chronically infected prior to pregnancy, with or without reinfection during at various stages of gestation [22].

## CONCLUDING REMARKS

Therefore, congenital *T. gondii* infection was common when ewes were chronically infected prior to pregnancy, with or without reinfection during at various stages of gestation

## CONSENT FOR PUBLICATION

Not applicable.

## CONFLICT OF INTEREST

The authors declare no conflict of interest, financial or otherwise.

## ACKNOWLEDGEMENTS

Declared none

## REFERENCES

[1]     Tenter AM, Heckeroth AR, Weiss LM. *Toxoplasma gondii*: from animals to humans. Int J Parasitol 2000; 30(12-13): 1217-58.
        [http://dx.doi.org/10.1016/S0020-7519(00)00124-7] [PMID: 11113252]

[2]     MONLUX WS: Toxoplasma infection in animals. Cornell Vet 1942; 32: 316-6.

[3]     Buxton D, Maley SW, Wright SE, Rodger S, Bartley P, Innes EA. *Toxoplasma gondii* and ovine toxoplasmosis: new aspects of an old story. Vet Parasitol 2007; 149(1-2): 25-8.
        [http://dx.doi.org/10.1016/j.vetpar.2007.07.003] [PMID: 17686585]

[4]     Mainar RC, de la Cruz C, Asensio A, Domínguez L, Vázquez-Boland JA. Prevalence of agglutinating antibodies to *Toxoplasma gondii* in small ruminants of the Madrid region, Spain, and identification of factors influencing seropositivity by multivariate analysis. Vet Res Commun 1996; 20(2): 153-9.
        [http://dx.doi.org/10.1007/BF00385636] [PMID: 8711895]

[5]     Wyss R, Sager H, Müller N, *et al.* The occurrence of *Toxoplasma gondii* and *Neospora caninum* as regards meat hygiene. Schweiz Arch Tierheilkd 2000; 142(3): 95-108.
        [PMID: 10748708]

[6]     Pereira-Bueno J, Quintanilla-Gozalo A, Pérez-Pérez V, Alvarez-García G, Collantes-Fernández E, Ortega-Mora LM. Evaluation of ovine abortion associated with *Toxoplasma gondii* in Spain by different diagnostic techniques. Vet Parasitol 2004; 121(1-2): 33-43.
        [http://dx.doi.org/10.1016/j.vetpar.2004.02.004] [PMID: 15110401]

[7]     Lopes AP, Vilares A, Neto F, *et al.* Genotyping Characterization of *Toxoplasma gondii* in Cattle, Sheep, Goats and Swine from the North of Portugal. Iran J Parasitol 2015; 10(3): 465-72.
        [PMID: 26622302]

[8]     Dubey JP. Toxoplasmosis in sheep--the last 20 years. Vet Parasitol 2009; 163(1-2): 1-14.
        [http://dx.doi.org/10.1016/j.vetpar.2009.02.026] [PMID: 19395175]

[9]     Armand B, Solhjoo K, Shabani-Kordshooli M, Davami MH, Sadeghi M. Toxoplasma infection in sheep from south of Iran monitored by serological and molecular methods; risk assessment to meat consumers. Vet World 2016; 9(8): 850-5.
        [http://dx.doi.org/10.14202/vetworld.2016.850-855] [PMID: 27651673]

[10]    Sharif M, Sarvi Sh, Shokri A, *et al. Toxoplasma gondii* infection among sheep and goats in Iran: a systematic review and meta-analysis. Parasitol Res 2015; 114(1): 1-16.
        [http://dx.doi.org/10.1007/s00436-014-4176-2] [PMID: 25378258]

[11]    dos Santos TR, Nunes CM, Luvizotto MC, *et al.* Detection of *Toxoplasma gondii* oocysts in environmental samples from public schools. Vet Parasitol 2010; 171(1-2): 53-7.
        [http://dx.doi.org/10.1016/j.vetpar.2010.02.045] [PMID: 20347524]

[12]    Hartley WJ. Experimental transmission of toxoplasmosis in sheep. N Z Vet J 1961; 9: 1-6.
        [http://dx.doi.org/10.1080/00480169.1961.33404]

[13]    Beverley JK, Watson WA, Spence JB. The pathology of the foetus in ovine abortion due to toxoplasmosis. Vet Rec 1971; 88(7): 174-8.
        [http://dx.doi.org/10.1136/vr.88.7.174] [PMID: 5102171]

[14]    Watson WA, Beverley JK. Ovine abortion due to experimental toxoplasmosis. Vet Rec 1971; 88(2): 42-5.
        [http://dx.doi.org/10.1136/vr.88.2.42] [PMID: 5100591]

[15]    Miller JK, Blewett DA, Buxton D. Clinical and serological response of pregnant gimmers to

experimentally induced toxoplasmosis. Vet Rec 1982; 111(6): 124-6.
[http://dx.doi.org/10.1136/vr.111.6.124] [PMID: 7123831]

[16]   Blewett DA, Miller JK, Buxton D. Response of immune and susceptible ewes to infection with *Toxoplasma gondii*. Vet Rec 1982; 111(9): 175-8.
[http://dx.doi.org/10.1136/vr.111.9.175] [PMID: 6890266]

[17]   Duncanson P, Terry RS, Smith JE, Hide G. High levels of congenital transmission of *Toxoplasma gondii* in a commercial sheep flock. Int J Parasitol 2001; 31(14): 1699-703.
[http://dx.doi.org/10.1016/S0020-7519(01)00282-X] [PMID: 11730799]

[18]   Morley EK, Williams RH, Hughes JM, *et al.* Significant familial differences in the frequency of abortion and *Toxoplasma gondii* infection within a flock of Charollais sheep. Parasitology 2005; 131(Pt 2): 181-5.
[http://dx.doi.org/10.1017/S0031182005007614] [PMID: 16145934]

[19]   Williams RH, Morley EK, Hughes JM, *et al.* High levels of congenital transmission of *Toxoplasma gondii* in longitudinal and cross-sectional studies on sheep farms provides evidence of vertical transmission in ovine hosts. Parasitology 2005; 130(Pt 3): 301-7.
[http://dx.doi.org/10.1017/S0031182004006614] [PMID: 15796013]

[20]   Morley EK, Williams RH, Hughes JM, *et al.* Evidence that primary infection of Charollais sheep with *Toxoplasma gondii* may not prevent foetal infection and abortion in subsequent lambings. Parasitology 2008; 135(2): 169-73.
[http://dx.doi.org/10.1017/S0031182007003721] [PMID: 17922930]

[21]   Rodger SM, Maley SW, Wright SE, *et al.* Role of endogenous transplacental transmission in toxoplasmosis in sheep. Vet Rec 2006; 159(23): 768-72.
[PMID: 17142624]

[22]   Dos Santos TR, Faria GD, Guerreiro BM, *et al.* Congenital Toxoplasmosis in Chronically Infected and Subsequently Challenged Ewes. PLoS One 2016; 11(10): e0165124.
[http://dx.doi.org/10.1371/journal.pone.0165124] [PMID: 27788185]

# CHAPTER 6

# Congenital Toxoplasmosis in Pigs

## João Luis Garcia[*]

*Protozoology laboratory, Preventive Veterinary Medicine Department, Londrina State University, Londrina, PR, Brazil*

**Abstract:** *Toxoplasma gondii* is a protozoan parasite distributed worldwide. It is an obligatory intracellular parasite which can infect a wide variety of vertebrates and different host cells. Usually, *T. gondii* infect pigs without causing any clinical signs. However, although rare, it may provoke disease, presenting fever, anorexia, depression and abortion. Pork is considered the main infection source for humans, and the risk of acquiring infection through the consumption of raw or undercooked meat, which is common in many regions, shows that the control of swine toxoplasmosis plays an important role in the epidemiology of the disease. This chapter discusses aspects related to the parasite-host relationship between *T. gondii* and pigs, such as epidemiology, natural (congenital) and experimental infections, diagnosis, vaccines and prevention.

**Keywords:** Apicomplexa, Coccidia, Congenital infection, Epidemiology, Piglets, Protozoa infection, Protozoa parasites, Swine, Tissue cysts, *Toxoplasma gondii*, Toxoplasmatidae, Toxoplasmosis infection, Vertical transmission.

## INTRODUCTION

Pigs are considered the main infection source of toxoplasmosis to humans in the United States [1]. The occurrence and distribution of *T. gondii* have been related to climatic conditions and influenced by temperature, rainfall and humidity. The animal's age, breed, environmental conditions and management in general are the main determinants of prevalence of antibodies against *T. gondii*. Transmission of *T. gondii* to pigs occurs primarily by drinking water, food and soil contaminated with oocysts eliminated in the feces of cats and by eating tissue cysts containing the parasite. Young cats have been identified as the primary source of transmission of *T. gondii* to swine [2].

Natural toxoplasmosis in pigs was first diagnosed in the United States by Farrell *et al.* [3] in a herd that had increased mortality in all age groups. After this

---

[*] **Corresponding author João Luis Garcia:** Protozoology laboratory, Preventive Veterinary Medicine Department, Londrina State University, Londrina, PR, Brazil; Tel/Fax: (43) 3371-4765; E-mail: jlgarcia@uel.br

finding, serological studies have demonstrated the high prevalence of *T. gondii* in Europe and the US [4].

The prevalence of anti-*T.gondii* antibodies in swine were previously described [5, 6]. Several serological studies, in pigs of different categories, showed a wide variation in the prevalence of toxoplasmosis, which ranged from 4 to 37.8% [7 - 14]. These wide variations may be explained by the different regional-geographical factors of the different production systems in each country [11].

The high levels of production and consumption of pork, combined with high spread and prevalence of *T. gondii*, also associated with the fact that cysts can remain viable in muscles of infected pigs for up to 875 days [15] and are not detectable in inspection at slaughter [16], make this food potentially hazardous in the transmission of toxoplasmosis to humans, when eating raw or undercooked pork.

A study conducted by Navarro *et al.* [17, 18] emphasized the importance of pork as an infection source of *T. gondii*. Likewise, Dias *et al.* [18] analyzed 149 samples of fresh pork sausages obtained from Londrina region, and after bioassay in mice, 13 (8.7%) of the samples were positive, and in one of them, it was possible to isolate *T. gondii*. For this reason, the control of swine toxoplasmosis plays an important role in the epidemiology of disease [19]. Tests available for detection of the disease in swine, as bioassays and serological tests, cannot be done on a routine basis during meat inspection. Thus, the assessment of infection rates together with efforts to reduce infection by improving management of the property, would be one of the measures to reduce the potential risk of contaminated pork consumption with *T. gondii* [20].

*T. gondii* can be controlled by sanitary education, management of animals, including livestock and cats, treatment, and vaccination. Treatment with drugs are used for diminishing clinical signs, however there are no drugs able to kill the parasite inside of the host cells. Additionally, there is no commercial vaccine available for pigs [21].

## TOXOPLASMOSIS IN PIGS

The *T. gondii* infection in pigs rarely shows clinical signs, and abortion in sows is not common, though it still may happen [5, 22 - 24]. The severity of the disease is related to age, sex hormones, pregnancy, immunological status, host nutritional condition, strain (including differences among strains) [25], parasite stages, and concomitant infections [19]. The mechanisms involved in the protection against infection are the components of the humoral and cellular immune response [21]

Host response to *T. gondii* is related to natural (innate) and acquired (adaptive) resistance. The differences between virulent strains of the parasite are important in host resistance, with molecular basis for these differences still unknown. Three clonal lineages of *T. gondii* are recognized and correlated with the virulence of the parasite. Lineage type 1 is associated with virulence in the acute phase in mice, type 2 strain is related to inducing chronic phase and the type 3 strain is less virulent to mice [26].

After the acute phase, the host develops adequate immunity, which is durable and protective against reinfection, while in the chronic phase, the parasite is maintained in tissue cysts. High titers of specific antibodies in the presence of complement as well as antibody dependent cellular cytotoxicity of antibodies can destroy the extracellular parasites, blocking the host cell invasion since the maximum production of antibodies coincides with the disappearance of viable tachyzoites [27].

## NATURAL INFECTION

Signs of spontaneous toxoplasmosis are uncommon in pigs, however, there are reports since 1950´s [3]. In Brasil, the first evidence of clinical toxoplasmosis in pigs was reported in Minas Gerais state in 1959 [28].

The natural toxoplasmosis in pigs was first diagnosed in the United States by Farrell and co-workers [3], on a farm in Ohio, during which the animals developed symptoms including weakness, cough, motor incoordination, tremors and diarrhea, leading to death in 50% of these. In addition, there were stillbirths, premature births and perinatal death.

In Japan, Moriwaki and co-workers [29] described congenital infection with signs of abortion and stillbirth. The authors described piglets with paralysis and many organs of these animals with lesions suggesting presence of *T. gondii.*

In Ontario, Canada, Hunter [23] described an abortion in a sow being associated with *T. gondii.* The aborted foetus was near to the end term, the sow showed a high level of antibodies against *T. gondii*, and sections of the placenta were also reported to be infected.

Chang and co-workers [30] described toxoplasmosis abortion in pigs from farms in Taiwan during which degenerative lesions associated with tachyzoites in placenta and fetal tissues were described.

In Brazil, Giraldi and co-workers [31] described neonatal toxoplasmosis in two aborted fetuses, six stillborn, and 10 neonatal piglets, in which tachyzoites of

*T. gondii* were observed in histological sections of the brain, heart, lung, liver, retina and spleens of infected piglets.

Venturini and co-workers [32], in Argentina, detected antibodies against *T. gondii* in 15 out of 738 fetal fluids from piglets derived from three swine farms by using the indirect immunofluorescence assay (IFA) and the modified agglutination test (MAT) for antibody detection.

Kim and co-workers [24] investigated an outbreak of porcine abortion associated with *T. gondii* in Jeju Island, Korea, during which the affected sows showed elevated fever, anorexia, vomiting, depression, recumbency, prostration, abortion, and a few deaths.

## EXPERIMENTAL INFECTION

Experimental infection with *T. gondii* in pigs has been conducted for different purposes, usually, to assess the virulence of isolates, distribution of cysts in the tissues and protection against experimental challenge in vaccinated animals.

The RH strain of *T. gondii* is the most commonly used and studied in laboratories. Much of the knowledge about the biology of this parasite was determined by the characterization of the RH strain [25]. This strain was isolated in 1939 by Sabin [33] from a case of congenital fatal encephalitis due to *T. gondii*. Since then, this strain has been propagated *in vitro* in cell cultures and *in vivo* in mice in several laboratories worldwide. However, there are differences between the RH strains maintained in different laboratories, and this variation is due to genetic differences probably caused by 50 years of cultivation and passages in mice [25].

In addition to the genetic differences between the RH strains, the inoculation route may also influence the pathogenicity in the affected animal. Dubey and co-workers [34] inoculated pigs with $10^5$ tachyzoites of the RH strain by the intramuscular and intravenous routes, the animals were either febrile or developed symptoms and died, respectively. Cysts of *T. gondii* were demonstrated in pigs at 42 and 64 dpi with the RH strain inoculated either subcutaneously or through intramuscular route [35]. Similarly, Garcia and co-workers [36] did not observe clinical signs in pigs infected intramuscularly with $7 \times 10^7$ tachyzoites of the RH strain. This strain does not present as persistent in pig tissues as it was found in the liver lesions (4-14 days PI) of the inoculated animals, indicating that this organ can serve as a site for the multiplication and / or elimination of *T. gondii* [34]. Pinckney and co-workers [1] described conjunctivitis, chorioretinitis and ocular ulcerations at days 7, 9, 14 and 60 after infection *via* the intravenous route with the RH strain.

Vidotto and co-workers [37] inoculated $10^4$ oocysts of the AS-28 strain in pregnant sows and observed clinical signs such as hyperthermia, anorexia, nasal discharge, tachypnea, lacrimation, prostration and abortion from the 4th day after infection.

Dubey and co-workers [35] after vaccinating pigs with the RH strain, challenged the animals with oocysts from a mixture of five strains of *T. gondii*. Three to eight days after the challenge, the animals demonstrated fever, diarrhea and anorexia. Furthermore, one animal that received the dose of $10^5$ oocysts became severely ill and had to be euthanized nine days after challenge, while *T. gondii* was isolated from multiple tissues such as the tongue, heart and brain of the pigs by bioassay in mice 42 days after the challenge.

Bekner da Silva and co-workers [38] infected pigs by the intravenous (IV) route and observed only hyperthermia. These authors used $10^6$ of living tachyzoites of the RH strain, LIV strain (isolated from swine), CPL-I (isolated from goat) and HV-III (dog isolated).

A study with TS-4 mutant strain (thermo sensitive strain) revealed that pigs inoculated either by the IV or subcutaneous (SC) route with $3 \times 10^5$ of live tachyzoites of TS4 did not develop clinical signs and TS-4 strain was not isolated from tissues of infected animals. In addition, the animals had low antibody titers by MAT in both inoculation routes. Moreover, the authors reported that age was not a factor in the susceptibility of pigs inoculated with the strain TS-4, since in that study animals were inoculated at three days of age. In the same experiment, the animals were submitted to a challenge with $8 \times 10^4$ oocysts of the GT-1 strain from which the authors found that the TS-4 strain does not prevent the formation of tissue cysts in pigs, but can reduce the number of tissue cysts in animals inoculated by the SC route and protect against clinical disease.

Jungersen and co-workers [39] demonstrated that a moderate dose of the NED strain (isolated from human with congenital toxoplasmosis) appeared to be more virulent for animals than the strains originating from swine (SSI 119 and P14) or the strain isolated from the myocardium of a fox (FOX2). However, the strain isolated (O14) from a sheep that was aborted demonstrated lower responses to the parameters used to characterize the virulence of *T. gondii*. In that experiment, $10^4$ tachyzoites were inoculated IV in piglets (6-7 weeks) to evaluate virulence. All pigs with the exception of the group that received the O14 showed a slight increase in temperature six to eight days post-inoculation (PI). Another group of piglets which received a dose of $10^6$ tachyzoites of the SSI119 strain become clinically ill with fever for four days PI, leading to the death of one pig on the sixth day PI and temperature variations until the 17th day PI.

In order to assess protection against the formation of tissue cyst, Garcia and co-workers [36] vaccinated pigs with crude rhoptries of *T. gondii* incorporated into immune stimulating complexes (ISCOM). After challenging with 4 x $10^4$ oocysts of the VEG strain, partial protection and a reduced production of tissue cysts in vaccinated animals compared to control animals were observed. The inoculated animals showed clinical signs from four to seven days, initially with ocular secretions followed by cough, anorexia, prostration and high fever. These animals recovered eight days after inoculation, and most muscle and brain tissue samples were positive in the mice bioassay.

The differences in pathogenicity of the various strains of *T. gondii* indicate that the virulence of the strains may vary with relation to the genotype. These differences may be related to the adaptation in the host or additional modifications associated with inherent proliferative potential of the strains in culture media [39]. This reinforces the idea that virulence is not an intrinsic factor of the parasite, but is dependent on the host-parasite interaction. These differences observed in the virulence of *T. gondii* strains in different hosts indicate that other genetic parameters, in addition to those described by Howe and Sibley and co-workers [25], determine the pathogenicity for a given host [39].

## DIAGNOSIS

The diagnosis of porcine toxoplasmosis is based on clinical signals (when they occur), direct diagnosis of the parasite or indirectly by detecting antibodies by serological tests. Direct diagnosis can be performed by bioassay in animals (primarily in mice and cats), which is the predominant method used to detect tissue cysts. Bioassay in cats is highly sensitive, and is considered the gold standard for the detection of *T. gondii* [40]. However, this procedure has the disadvantages of presenting risks to the applicant, is laborious and very expensive.

The polymerase chain reaction (PCR) is a powerful molecular technique that detects parasite in various body fluids, tissues and blood. This method has good sensitivity, high specificity, and is a technique, which can be performed quickly [41]. Jauregui and co-workers [42] developed a real-time PCR assay to detect *T. gondii* in tissues of pigs and suggest that this technique can complement or even replace the bioassay techniques. However, Garcia and co-workers [43] observed a better performance in mouse bioassay for the detection of *T. gondii* in the tissues of pigs when compared with PCR.

Histopathology is not efficient in detecting cysts of *T. gondii* in large animal tissue samples [43]. This can be explained by the fact that pigs and others large animals have less than one cyst/50g of tissue [15]. Immunohistochemistry is more efficient during the acute phase of infection, and it is capable of detecting tachyzoites and bradyzoites in tissues [43].

The occurrence of antibodies against *T. gondii* is associated with the presence of viable parasites in either organs or tissues of pig [44]. Several serological tests may be used for the detection of anti-*T. gondii* antibodies, including the Sabin-Feldman (SF) or dye test, immunofluorescence assay (IFA), latex agglutination (LA), IHA, ELISA and the modified agglutination test (MAT) [45, 46]. ELISA and IFA are the assays that can distinguish between IgG and IgM antibodies, while MAT cannot distinguish between IgG and IgM. However, the production of IgM in swine is short-lived, and therefore may not be a good method to evaluate the time of infection [47].

SF is difficult to apply, is a biohazard because of the use of live tachyzoites as antigens, and is rarely used in the serodiagnosis of animals. MAT has good specificity when compared with sera from pigs experimentally infected with viruses, helminths and protozoa as *Neospora caninum* and *Sarcocystis miescheriana* [48].

When compared with other serologic assays, ELISA has several advantages, such as the interpretation of the results is not subjective, is more appropriate for large-scale use, and is cheaper than the MAT [49]. Moreover, the indirect ELISA showed better performance than MAT in the detection of antibodies against *T. gondii* in serum derived from experimentally and naturally infected pigs [20, 50]. However, cross reactivity resulting in false positive results is one of the most important problems when soluble antigens of *T. gondii* are used in indirect ELISA [44]. However, this does not occur with the dye test and IFAT [51], and MAT does not react with *S. miescheriana* [48].

IFA detects antibodies during the acute phase of infection, by recognizing membrane surface antigens of intact tachyzoites, while antibodies in ELISA are detected during the chronic stage of infection [46].

MAT and ELISA were evaluated to investigate *T. gondii* infection in naturally infected pigs and these tests presented sensitivity and specificity of 82.9% and 90.2% respectively for MAT and 72.9% and 85.9% for ELISA [52]. However, an ELISA assay using crude rhoptries as antigen (r-ELISA) to detect antibodies against *T. gondii* in experimentally infected pigs demonstrated a higher prevalence (76%), sensitivity (98.5%), negative predictive value (95%), and accuracy (98.8%) than MAT, additionally, the Kappa agreements between tests were calculated, and the best results were obtained by r-ELISA x IFAT (k=0.86) [46]. However, the conditions of both studies were different, the first study consisted of naturally infected pigs and the mouse bioassay was used as the gold standard, whereas the second investigation contained experimentally infected pigs and IFAT was used as the gold standard.

## VACCINES

The first generation of vaccines was elaborated with live, live attenuated, or inactivated antigens, second generation consisted of the subunit vaccines (single protein purified or recombinant), and finally third generation immunogens is based on genetic vaccines [53]. Since live and inactivated vaccines are considered as foreign by the immune system, they active a series of reactive lymphocytes and induce antibody production which can block infection [54].

An important factor in *T. gondii* infection is that, the main route of infection of the host is oral, so local immunity in the gut *via* lymphocytes (mainly intraepithelial lymphocytes presenting $CD8^+$ activities) and IgA is of fundamental importance for host resistance to the parasite [55]. However, after the initial infection by the sporozoites, the parasites are transformed into tachyzoites, the rapidly dividing form of the parasite, thus the sporoSAG protein is non-immunogenic during natural infection [56].

Tissue cysts in pork can persist for more than two years and it is one of the most important sources of *T. gondii* infections in human [35, 57]; consequently, an adequate vaccine to control *T. gondii* in pigs should be able to avoid tissue cysts formation.

Studies using live RH strain showed some protection against tissue cyst formation [1, 35, 36], but these results were not enough to indicate that this can be used as a live vaccine in pigs considering the fact that there are pathogenicity differences between RH strain in pigs [58]. The RH strain was not persistent in pig tissues 64 days after infection (dai) [35]. In a study in our laboratory, Bugni and co-workers [59] observed that the RH strain was not able to form tissue cysts 69 dai. The RH strain is the most widely investigated and used strain of *T. gondii* in laboratories. This strain was isolated from a child with toxoplasmic encephalitis in 1939 [33] and since then has been maintained in mice and cellular culture.

A vaccine study using crude *T. gondii* antigens incorporated in ISCOM by subcutaneous route in pigs did not isolate, by mouse bioassay, tissue cysts from vaccinated animals [60]. Garcia and co-workers [36] used rhoptry proteins incorporated in ISCOM to prevent tissue cyst formation in pigs challenged with sporulated oocysts of the VEG strain. The results indicated that rhoptry vaccine conferred partial protection during the chronic phase of the disease.

Pigs were immunized intradermally with a cocktail DNA vaccine encoded with GRA1 and GRA7 dense granules proteins [61]. The authors described that this vaccine was able to elicit a strong humoral and Type 1 cellular immune response in vaccinated animals. Unfortunately, the results relative to tissue cysts burden evaluation were inconsistent; nevertheless, this study was important because an immune response was elicited in pigs through a DNA vaccine.

Verhelst and co-workers [62] demonstrated that GRA7 and MIC3 were able to induce adequate humoral immune response in pigs experimentally challenged with tissue cysts of *T. gondii*. Cunha and co-workers [63] evaluated the protection obtained against tissue cyst formation in pigs immunized intranasally with a crude rhoptry protein preparation of *T. gondii* plus Quil-A, and revealed that the vaccinated and challenged group had 41.6% protection against tissue cyst formation, compared with 6.5% protection in the control group.

Excreted–secreted antigens (ESAs, the proteins that are discharged from organelles of the parasite during invasion of host cells) from *T. gondii* mixed with Freund's adjuvant were used as a vaccine in pigs to evaluate the humoral and cellular immune responses and protection against an intraperitoneal challenge with $10^7$ tachyzoites of the GJS strain [64]. The authors described a cellular immune response associated with the production of IFN-$\gamma$ and IL-4, and a humoral response mainly against antigens with molecular masses between 34 and 116 kDa. Following the challenge, the immunized pigs were asymptomatic except for an increase in temperature, while the control animals developed a higher fever and clinical signs indicative of toxoplasmosis. They also described a reduction in tissue cyst formation in the muscles of the vaccinated animals.

## CONTROL STRATEGIES

The strategies used to control toxoplasmosis in pigs need to focus on cats, food and drinking water. The control of rats and mouse in a farm should be assured because the dry food that is available to farm animals is also attractive to rodents and consequently cats. Additionally, predation of rats by pigs is also common. Cats should receive only dry food or foods that have undergone heat treatment (>67 °C).

Epidemiological studies conducted in northern Paraná, in pig herds, showed the constant presence of domestic cats and rodents in piggeries and pastures next to the house of the properties, which could explain the high rates of seropositive animals [10]. Sporadic outbreaks can be controlled with chemotherapy (sulfonamides) and prophilactic measures.

## CONSENT FOR PUBLICATION

Not applicable.

## CONFLICT OF INTEREST

The authors declare no conflict of interest, financial or otherwise.

## ACKNOWLEDGEMENTS

Declared none

## REFERENCES

[1]     Pinckney RD, Lindsay DS, Blagburn BL, Boosinger TR, McLaughlin SA, Dubey JP. Evaluation of the safety and efficacy of vaccination of nursing pigs with living tachyzoites of two strains of *Toxoplasma gondii*. J Parasitol 1994; 80(3): 438-48.
[http://dx.doi.org/10.2307/3283415] [PMID: 8195946]

[2]     Mateus-Pinilla NE, Dubey JP, Choromanski L, Weigel RM. A field trial of the effectiveness of a feline *Toxoplasma gondii* vaccine in reducing *T. gondii* exposure for swine. J Parasitol 1999; 85(5): 855-60.
[http://dx.doi.org/10.2307/3285821] [PMID: 10577720]

[3]     Farrell RL, Docton FL, Chamberlain DM, Cole CR. Toxoplasmosis. I. Toxoplasma isolated from swine. Am J Vet Res 1952; 13(47): 181-5.
[PMID: 14924136]

[4]     Tenter AM, Heckeroth AR, Weiss LM. *Toxoplasma gondii*: from animals to humans. Int J Parasitol 2000; 30(12-13): 1217-58.
[http://dx.doi.org/10.1016/S0020-7519(00)00124-7] [PMID: 11113252]

[5]     Dubey JP. Toxoplasmosis in pigs--the last 20 years. Vet Parasitol 2009; 164(2-4): 89-103.
[http://dx.doi.org/10.1016/j.vetpar.2009.05.018] [PMID: 19559531]

[6]     Dubey JP. A review of toxoplasmosis in pigs. Vet Parasitol 1986; 19(3-4): 181-223.
[http://dx.doi.org/10.1016/0304-4017(86)90070-1] [PMID: 3518210]

[7]     Carletti RTF. Prevalência da infecção por *Toxoplasma gondii* em suínos abatidos no Estado do Paraná, Brasil. Semin Cienc Agrar 2005; 26(4): 563-8.
[http://dx.doi.org/10.5433/1679-0359.2005v26n4p563]

[8]     Suaréz-Aranda F, Galisteo AJ, Hiramoto RM, *et al.* The prevalence and avidity of *Toxoplasma gondii* IgG antibodies in pigs from Brazil and Peru. Vet Parasitol 2000; 91(1-2): 23-32.
[http://dx.doi.org/10.1016/S0304-4017(00)00249-1] [PMID: 10889357]

[9]     Soroepidemiologia e fatores associados a transmissão do *Toxoplasma gondii* em suínos do norte do Paraná. Arch Vet Sci 2003; 8: 27-34.

[10]    Vidotto O, Navarro IT, Giraldi IT, *et al.* Estudos epidemiológicos da toxoplasmose em suínos da região de Londrina - PR. Semina 1990; 11(1): 53-9.

[11]    Garcia JLN IT, Ogawa L, *et al.* Seroprevalence of *Toxoplasma gondii* in swine, bovine, ovine and equine, and their correlation with human, felines and canines, from farms in north region of paraná state, Brazil. Ciência Rural 1999; 29(1): 91-7.

[12]    Samico Fernandes EF, Samico Fernandes MF, Kim PC, *et al.* Prevalence of *Toxoplasma gondii* in slaughtered pigs in the state of Pernambuco, Brazil. J Parasitol 2012; 98(3): 690-1.
[http://dx.doi.org/10.1645/GE-3032.1] [PMID: 22263703]

[13]    Azevedo SS, Pena HF, Alves CJ, *et al.* Prevalence of anti-*Toxoplasma gondii* and anti-Neospora caninum antibodies in swine from Northeastern Brazil. Rev Bras Parasitol Vet 2010; 19(2): 80-4.
[http://dx.doi.org/10.1590/S1984-29612010000200002] [PMID: 20624342]

[14]    Cavalcante GT, Aguiar DM, Chiebao D, *et al.* Seroprevalence of *Toxoplasma gondii* antibodies in cats and pigs from rural Western Amazon, Brazil. J Parasitol 2006; 92(4): 863-4.

[http://dx.doi.org/10.1645/GE-830R.1] [PMID: 16995406]

[15] Dubey JP. Long-term persistence of *Toxoplasma gondii* in tissues of pigs inoculated with *T. gondii* oocysts and effect of freezing on viability of tissue cysts in pork. Am J Vet Res 1988; 49(6): 910-3.
[PMID: 3400928]

[16] Hirvelä-Koski V. Evaluation of ELISA for the detection of Toxoplasma antibodies in swine sera. Acta Vet Scand 1990; 31(4): 413-22.
[PMID: 2099619]

[17] Navarro IT, Vidotto O, Giraldi N, Mitsuka R. [Resistance of *Toxoplasma gondii* to sodium chloride and condiments in pork sausage]. Bol Oficina Sanit Panam 1992; 112(2): 138-43. [Resistance of *Toxoplasma gondii* to sodium chloride and condiments in pork sausage].
[PMID: 1531110]

[18] Dias RA, Navarro IT, Ruffolo BB, Bugni FM, Castro MV, Freire RL. *Toxoplasma gondii* in fresh pork sausage and seroprevalence in butchers from factories in Londrina, Paraná State, Brazil. Rev Inst Med Trop São Paulo 2005; 47(4): 185-9.
[http://dx.doi.org/10.1590/S0036-46652005000400002] [PMID: 16138196]

[19] Dubey JP. Toxoplasmosis. J Am Vet Med Assoc 1994; 205(11): 1593-8.
[PMID: 7730132]

[20] Gamble HR, Dubey JP, Lambillotte DN. Comparison of a commercial ELISA with the modified agglutination test for detection of Toxoplasma infection in the domestic pig. Vet Parasitol 2005; 128(3-4): 177-81.
[http://dx.doi.org/10.1016/j.vetpar.2004.11.019] [PMID: 15740853]

[21] Garcia JL. Vaccination concepts against *Toxoplasma gondii*. Expert Rev Vaccines 2009; 8(2): 215-25.
[http://dx.doi.org/10.1586/14760584.8.2.215] [PMID: 19196201]

[22] Li X, Wang Y, Yu F, Li T, Zhang D. An outbreak of lethal toxoplasmosis in pigs in the Gansu province of China. Journal of veterinary diagnostic investigation: official publication of the American Association of Veterinary Laboratory Diagnosticians. Inc 2010; 22(3): 442-4.

[23] Hunter B. Isolated, spontaneous Toxoplasma abortion in a young sow. Can Vet J 1979; 20(4): 116.
[PMID: 427708]

[24] Kim JH, Kang KI, Kang WC, *et al.* Porcine abortion outbreak associated with *Toxoplasma gondii* in Jeju Island, Korea. J Vet Sci 2009; 10(2): 147-51.
[http://dx.doi.org/10.4142/jvs.2009.10.2.147] [PMID: 19461210]

[25] Howe DK, Sibley LD. *Toxoplasma gondii*: analysis of different laboratory stocks of the RH strain reveals genetic heterogeneity. Exp Parasitol 1994; 78(2): 242-5.
[http://dx.doi.org/10.1006/expr.1994.1024] [PMID: 7907030]

[26] Howe DK, Summers BC, Sibley LD. Acute virulence in mice is associated with markers on chromosome VIII in *Toxoplasma gondii*. Infect Immun 1996; 64(12): 5193-8.
[PMID: 8945565]

[27] Frenkel JK. Transmission of toxoplasmosis and the role of immunity in limiting transmission and illness. J Am Vet Med Assoc 1990; 196(2): 233-40.
[PMID: 2404921]

[28] JML S. Sobre um caso de toxoplasmose espontânea em suínos. Arch Vet Sci 1959; 12: 425-8.

[29] Moriwaki M, Hayashi S, Minami T, Ishitani R. Detection of congenital toxoplasmosis in piglet. Nippon Juigaku Zasshi 1976; 38(4): 377-81.
[http://dx.doi.org/10.1292/jvms1939.38.377] [PMID: 988417]

[30] Chang GN, Tsai SS, Kuo M, Dubey JP. Epidemiology of swine toxoplasmosis in Taiwan. Southeast Asian J Trop Med Public Health 1991; 22 (Suppl.): 111-4.
[PMID: 1822866]

[31]    Giraldi N, Freire RL, Navarro IT, Viotti NM, Bueno SG, Vidotto O. Estudo da toxoplasmose congenita natural em granjas de suinos em Londrina, PR. Arq Bras Med Vet Zootec 1996; 48: 83-90.

[32]    Venturini MC, Bacigalupe D, Venturini L, Machuca M, Perfumo CJ, Dubey JP. Detection of antibodies to *Toxoplasma gondii* in stillborn piglets in Argentina. Vet Parasitol 1999; 85(4): 331-4.
[http://dx.doi.org/10.1016/S0304-4017(99)00104-1] [PMID: 10488736]

[33]    Toxoplasmosis AB. recently recognized disease. Adv Pediatr 1942; 1: 1-54.

[34]    Dubey JP, Baker DG, Davis SW, Urban JF Jr, Shen SK. Persistence of immunity to toxoplasmosis in pigs vaccinated with a nonpersistent strain of *Toxoplasma gondii*. Am J Vet Res 1994; 55(7): 982-7.
[PMID: 7978639]

[35]    Dubey JP, Urban JF Jr, Davis SW. Protective immunity to toxoplasmosis in pigs vaccinated with a nonpersistent strain of *Toxoplasma gondii*. Am J Vet Res 1991; 52(8): 1316-9.
[PMID: 1928915]

[36]    Garcia JL, Gennari SM, Navarro IT, *et al.* Partial protection against tissue cysts formation in pigs vaccinated with crude rhoptry proteins of *Toxoplasma gondii*. Vet Parasitol 2005; 129(3-4): 209-17.
[http://dx.doi.org/10.1016/j.vetpar.2005.01.006] [PMID: 15845275]

[37]    Vidotto OC. A. J.; Balarin, M. R. S.; Rocha, M. A. Toxoplasmose experimental em porcas gestantes. I. Observacoes clinicas e hematológicas. Arq Bras Med Vet Zootec 1987; 39(4): 623-39.

[38]    Bekner Da Silva AC. R.; Navarro, I. T. Avaliação pela imunofluorescência indireta dos aspectos imunogênicos e antigênicos de diferentes amostras de *Toxoplasma gondii* inoculadas em suínos. Rev Bras Parasitol Vet 1994; 3(1): 17-22.

[39]    Jungersen G, Jensen L, Riber U, *et al.* Pathogenicity of selected *Toxoplasma gondii* isolates in young pigs. Int J Parasitol 1999; 29(8): 1307-19.
[http://dx.doi.org/10.1016/S0020-7519(99)00078-8] [PMID: 10576580]

[40]    Dubey JP, Frenkel JK. Feline toxoplasmosis from acutely infected mice and the development of Toxoplasma cysts. J Protozool 1976; 23(4): 537-46.
[http://dx.doi.org/10.1111/j.1550-7408.1976.tb03836.x] [PMID: 1003342]

[41]    de A Dos Santos CB, de Carvalho AC, Ragozo AM, *et al.* First isolation and molecular characterization of *Toxoplasma gondii* from finishing pigs from São Paulo State, Brazil. Vet Parasitol 2005; 131(3-4): 207-11.
[http://dx.doi.org/10.1016/j.vetpar.2005.04.039] [PMID: 15951111]

[42]    Jauregui LH, Higgins J, Zarlenga D, Dubey JP, Lunney JK. Development of a real-time PCR assay for detection of *Toxoplasma gondii* in pig and mouse tissues. J Clin Microbiol 2001; 39(6): 2065-71.
[http://dx.doi.org/10.1128/JCM.39.6.2065-2071.2001] [PMID: 11376036]

[43]    Garcia JL, Gennari SM, Machado RZ, Navarro IT. *Toxoplasma gondii*: detection by mouse bioassay, histopathology, and polymerase chain reaction in tissues from experimentally infected pigs. Exp Parasitol 2006; 113(4): 267-71.
[http://dx.doi.org/10.1016/j.exppara.2006.02.001] [PMID: 16545804]

[44]    Andrews CD, Dubey JP, Tenter AM, Webert DW. *Toxoplasma gondii* recombinant antigens H4 and H11: use in ELISAs for detection of toxoplasmosis in swine. Vet Parasitol 1997; 70(1-3): 1-11.
[http://dx.doi.org/10.1016/S0304-4017(96)01154-5] [PMID: 9195704]

[45]    Montoya F, Ramirez L, Loaiza A, Henao J, Murillo G. Prevalence of antibodies against *Toxoplasma gondii* in cattle and swine. Bol Oficina Sanit Panam 1981; 91(3): 219-27.
[PMID: 6459104]

[46]    Garcia JL, Navarro IT, Vidotto O, *et al. Toxoplasma gondii*: comparison of a rhoptry-ELISA with IFAT and MAT for antibody detection in sera of experimentally infected pigs. Exp Parasitol 2006; 113(2): 100-5.
[http://dx.doi.org/10.1016/j.exppara.2005.12.011] [PMID: 16458299]

[47] Lind P, Haugegaard J, Wingstrand A, Henriksen SA. The time course of the specific antibody response by various ELISAs in pigs experimentally infected with *Toxoplasma gondii*. Vet Parasitol 1997; 71(1): 1-15.
[http://dx.doi.org/10.1016/S0304-4017(97)00010-1] [PMID: 9231984]

[48] Dubey JP. Validation of the specificity of the modified agglutination test for toxoplasmosis in pigs. Vet Parasitol 1997; 71(4): 307-10.
[http://dx.doi.org/10.1016/S0304-4017(97)00016-2] [PMID: 9299699]

[49] Weigel RM, Dubey JP, Siegel AM, *et al.* Prevalence of antibodies to *Toxoplasma gondii* in swine in Illinois in 1992. J Am Vet Med Assoc 1995; 206(11): 1747-51.
[PMID: 7782249]

[50] Hill DE, Chirukandoth S, Dubey JP, Lunney JK, Gamble HR. Comparison of detection methods for *Toxoplasma gondii* in naturally and experimentally infected swine. Vet Parasitol 2006; 141(1-2): 9-17.
[http://dx.doi.org/10.1016/j.vetpar.2006.05.008] [PMID: 16815636]

[51] Lovgren K, Uggla A, Morein B. A new approach to the preparation of a *Toxoplasma gondii* membrane antigen for use in ELISA. Zentralblatt fur Veterinarmedizin Reihe B Journal of veterinary medicine Series B 1987; 34(4): 274-82.

[52] Dubey JP, Thulliez P, Weigel RM, Andrews CD, Lind P, Powell EC. Sensitivity and specificity of various serologic tests for detection of *Toxoplasma gondii* infection in naturally infected sows. Am J Vet Res 1995; 56(8): 1030-6.
[PMID: 8533974]

[53] Kalinna BH. DNA vaccines for parasitic infections. Immunol Cell Biol 1997; 75(4): 370-5.
[http://dx.doi.org/10.1038/icb.1997.58] [PMID: 9315480]

[54] Babiuk LA. Vaccination: a management tool in veterinary medicine. Vet J 2002; 164(3): 188-201.
[http://dx.doi.org/10.1053/tvjl.2001.0663] [PMID: 12505392]

[55] Jongert E, Verhelst D, Abady M, Petersen E, Gargano N. Protective Th1 immune responses against chronic toxoplasmosis induced by a protein-protein vaccine combination but not by its DNA-protein counterpart. Vaccine 2008; 26(41): 5289-95.
[http://dx.doi.org/10.1016/j.vaccine.2008.07.032] [PMID: 18675872]

[56] Crawford J, Lamb E, Wasmuth J, Grujic O, Grigg ME, Boulanger MJ. Structural and functional characterization of SporoSAG: a SAG2-related surface antigen from *Toxoplasma gondii*. J Biol Chem 2010; 285(16): 12063-70.
[http://dx.doi.org/10.1074/jbc.M109.054866] [PMID: 20164173]

[57] Dubey JP, Lunney JK, Shen SK, Kwok OC. Immunity to toxoplasmosis in pigs fed irradiated *Toxoplasma gondii* oocysts. J Parasitol 1998; 84(4): 749-52.
[http://dx.doi.org/10.2307/3284582] [PMID: 9714205]

[58] Lindsay DS, Blagburn BL, Dubey JP. Safety and results of challenge of weaned pigs given a temperature-sensitive mutant of *Toxoplasma gondii*. J Parasitol 1993; 79(1): 71-6.
[http://dx.doi.org/10.2307/3283280] [PMID: 8437061]

[59] Bugni FM, Da Cunha IA, De Araújo MA, *et al.* Action of β-glucan in pigs experimentally infected with *Toxoplasma gondii* tachyzoites. Rev Bras Parasitol Vet 2008; 17 (Suppl. 1): 249-59.
[PMID: 20059858]

[60] Freire RL. Bracarense APFRL, Gennari SM. Vaccination of pigs with *Toxoplasma gondii* antigens incorporated in immunostimulating complexes (iscoms). Arq Bras Med Vet Zootec 2003; 55(4): 388-96.
[http://dx.doi.org/10.1590/S0102-09352003000400002]

[61] Jongert E, Melkebeek V, De Craeye S, Dewit J, Verhelst D, Cox E. An enhanced GRA1-GRA7 cocktail DNA vaccine primes anti-Toxoplasma immune responses in pigs. Vaccine 2008; 26(8): 1025-31.

[http://dx.doi.org/10.1016/j.vaccine.2007.11.058] [PMID: 18221825]

[62]    Verhelst D, De Craeye S, Dorny P, *et al.* IFN-γ expression and infectivity of Toxoplasma infected tissues are associated with an antibody response against GRA7 in experimentally infected pigs. Vet Parasitol 2011; 179(1-3): 14-21.
[http://dx.doi.org/10.1016/j.vetpar.2011.02.015] [PMID: 21414723]

[63]    da Cunha IA, Zulpo DL, Bogado AL, *et al.* Humoral and cellular immune responses in pigs immunized intranasally with crude rhoptry proteins of *Toxoplasma gondii* plus Quil-A. Vet Parasitol 2012; 186(3-4): 216-21.
[http://dx.doi.org/10.1016/j.vetpar.2011.11.034] [PMID: 22137347]

[64]    Wang Y, Zhang D, Wang G, Yin H, Wang M. Immunization with excreted-secreted antigens reduces tissue cyst formation in pigs. Parasitol Res 2013; 112(11): 3835-42.
[http://dx.doi.org/10.1007/s00436-013-3571-4] [PMID: 23949245]

# CHAPTER 7

# Congenital Toxoplasmosis in Goats

**Helenara Machado da Silva**[1,*], **Jesaías Ismael da Costa**[1], **Alvimar José da Costa**[1] and **Katia Denise Saraiva Bresciani**[1,2]

[1] *UNESP, Universidade Estadual Paulista (Unesp), Faculdade de Ciências Agrárias e Veterinárias de Jaboticabal, Jaboticabal, São Paulo, Brasil*

[2] *UNESP, Universidade Estadual Paulista (Unesp), Faculdade de Medicina Veterinária de Araçatuba, Araçatuba, São Paulo, Brasil. Research ID E-7126-2012*

**Abstract:** Toxoplasmosis is a public health issue and an obstacle to the breeding of goats. This zoonosis results in great economic losses in human beings and production animals, being both infected from the food and water intake contaminated with *Toxoplasma gondii* oocysts and this parasite causes severe clinical consequences, among them reproductive problems. In caprines, the presence of antibodies against *T. gondii* is common in herds. For this reason, toxoplasmic reinfection in these animals can not be ruled out or neglected in animals naturally infected with *T. gondii*. In this way, the objective of this chapter is to describe the main aspects of congenital toxoplasmosis in pregnant goats, in different gestational stages, infected and reinfected with *T. gondii* and their offspring.

**Keywords:** Clinical disorders, Clinical signs, Congenital problems, Control, Diagnosis, Epidemiology, Infection toxoplasmosis, Pathogenesis, Pregnant goats, Prevention, Reinfection toxoplasmosis, Reproductive losses, Treatment.

## INTRODUCTION

Toxoplasmosis is a public health issue and an obstacle to the breeding of goats, since meat, milk and skin of this animal species are consumed by humans and are a source of income for farmers. Therefore, economic losses are due to several reproductive disorders such as abortion, neonatal mortality and birth defects.

## EPIDEMIOLOGY

Generally, goats are susceptible to parasitism by *T. gondii*, independently of the animal category and age group. The most common injuries affect the reproductive system and generate irreversible congenital defects. On the other hand, the death

---

\* **Corresponding author Helenara Machado da Silva:** UNESP, Universidade Estadual Paulista Júlio de Mesquita Filho, Faculdade de Ciências Agrárias e Veterinárias de Jaboticabal, Jaboticabal, São Paulo, Brasil; Tel/Fax: +55 16 99732.9132; E-mail: helenarasilva@yahoo.com.br

of young and adult female goats may occur due to recurrent complications of this disease [1, 2].

However, it was verified that adult and purebred female goats present a higher risk of infection by coccidia when compared to young and mixed breed animals [3, 4].

## PATHOGENESIS AND CLINICAL SIGNS

In caprines, *T. gondii* on invading the placenta causes focal necrosis with mineral deposition on cotyledons, which directly affects placental-fetal endocrine function [5, 6]. In fetuses, *T. gondii* has a tropism by the phagocytic-mononuclear system, which induces the formation of pseudocysts that reach the blood circulation and are mainly lodged in the central nervous system and ocular region [7].

The host immune response against the infectious stage of toxoplasmosis is complex [8] and involves two types of responses: cellular and humoral [9]. The cellular immune response secretes cytokines with different action potentials, including those which interact with receptors in the hypothalamus and increase the thermoregulatory fixed point, causing elevation of body temperature. Thus, fever is another symptom observed in animals infected with *T. gondii* and this occurs mostly in the first days after toxoplasmic infection [10].

Females parasitized by *T. gondii* may present embryonic reabsorption, abortion, mummification, stillbirth, birth of weak offspring, body deformities, as well as generate apparently normal animals infected with *T. gondii*. Regarding abortion, it can occur in goats at any time after the ninth day after toxoplasmic infection and is closely related to the type of infecting strain [11].

Goats infected with *T. gondii* during the first third of gestation (first 50 days) present fetal death with subsequent resorption, abortion, mummification and stillbirth or birth of weak or apparently normal offspring [6]. Therefore, toxoplasmosis severity is higher when maternal infection occurs in the first trimester of gestation [12].

When toxoplasmic infection occurs in the middle third of gestation (between 70 and 90 days), the chances of abortion and stillbirth increase [13 - 15], while at the end of gestation (> 110 days), deliveries occur normally and there is a probability of the offspring born infected by *T. gondii* [14 - 16].

For this reason, toxoplasmic reinfection in goats cannot be ruled out or neglected in animals naturally infected with *T. gondii*. In a study of pregnant goats experimentally infected with *T. gondii* challenged with heterologous strains

(strains ME49 and VEG), toxoplasmic reinfection with congenital defects along the gestational three-thirds was proven, and reproductive losses were also estimated as a consequence of this parasitism [17, 18].

Toxoplasmosis in pregnant goats is a reproductive disease and thus it is important to differentiate it from other diseases, such as: brucellosis, leptospirosis and neosporosis that affect the reproductive system of females, especially goats.

Humoral responses of IgG antibodies to *Toxoplasma* vary widely for the goat species, which may be recent showing less than 15 days of infection [19 - 21], and delayed by 21 days of contact with *T. gondii* [22].

Another issue concerns the variation of antibody titers, which determines the toxoplasmosis phase, wherein the level of antibodies against *Toxoplasma* greater than or equal to 1024 is indicative of newly acquired toxoplasmic infection and below this threshold is suggestive of chronic infection [23]. Chronic or previous phase is the most common form of toxoplasmosis [24] and is characterized by the presence of class G immunoglobulins.

Reinfected goats developed a humoral immune response against *T. gondii*, indicative of acute toxoplasmosis, at all gestational stages (40, 80 and 120 days of gestation). Transplacental transmission to the respective offspring was also verified, which presented antibodies against Toxoplasma and parasitism by *T. gondii* [17, 18].

It is important to emphasize that, the stabilization of the chronic phase of toxoplasmosis in goats, acquired before pregnancy, was confirmed by the maintenance of serological titers of IgG class antibodies below 1024 [23]. This protected pregnant females from reproductive problems, such as fetal resorption and abortion, during reinfection with *T. gondii* oocysts. Such findings are frequent when there is primo-infection during pregnancy [22, 25].

It is worth noting, however, that other reproductive consequences were observed after *T. gondii* reinfections: premature birth, stillbirth, body deformities and births of weak animals at all gestational stages (40, 80 and 120 days post-gestation). The reproductive disorders affected 57.14%, 75.00% and 16.66% of offspring reinfected with *T. gondii* at 40, 80 and 120 days of gestation, respectively [17, 18].

In goats infected with *T. gondii*, no problems were observed during deliveries, which occurred within the period considered normal for the species and the birth of apparently healthy offspring, although some offspring of *T. gondii*-infected goats presented antibodies against this protozoan.

Another issue concerns the placenta sinepiteliocorial type characteristic of ruminants [26], which presents, among many peculiarities, the non-transference of maternal antibodies, such as anti-Toxoplasma, to fetuses [1]. The presence of antibodies in fetuses is indicative of infection [27, 28].

Additionally, an important issue concerns the maternal-fetal immune response, within the sequence of events involving *T. gondii* infection. When the tachyzoites reach the gravid uterus, they infect the placenta, where they multiply and through the bloodstream they spread to the fetal tissues [29]. In the fetal organism, usually, the *T. gondii* DNA can be detected [30].

## DIAGNOSIS

The methods of diagnosis of toxoplasmosis by histopathology, bioassay and polymerase chain reaction (PCR) allow identifying tissue parasitism in goats, but increase the price of the diagnosis of toxoplasmosis to the breeder therefore, they are usually performed for research purposes.

## PREVENTION

As mentioned above, the diagnosis of caprine toxoplasmosis by different laboratory methods (histopathology, bioassay and PCR), although effective in confirmation of the zoonosis goat herd, often becomes impractical due to its adoption in sanitary management routine for goat farmers. Another issue involves the costs of treatment of this disease, in both veterinary medicine and public health.

Thus, the adoption of preventive and control measures, as well as health education, is the most adequate way to avoid toxoplasmosis in goat breeding and in the general population. It is also important to guide the population about the need to consume foods of vegetable origin and animals of suitable origin that have undergone accredited inspection services.

Among preventive measures for the ingestion of food for humans, some precautionary measures can be taken while consuming the raw leafy green vegetables: wash them under cold running drinking water, then immerse them in chlorine solution for ten minutes, after this period rinse them again in abundant drinking water, remove excess water, pack them in sanitized containers and keep refrigerated until consumption [31].

In the case of products of animal origin, attention must be paid regarding dairy and fresh meat products, widely used in the preparation of fresh cheeses and sausages, respectively. Such raw materials (meat and milk) must be manufactured following good management practices, including hygiene at milking [32], and cooling the meat after slaughter [31]. Several studies have pointed out that the most frequent route of transmission of toxoplasmosis to humans is the ingestion of cysts through animal products, especially when they are ingested raw or without appropriate heat treatment [33 - 38].

In addition, *T. gondii* contamination was verified in the products of goat origin, both the milk [37, 39 - 44] and the musculature of animals [40, 45].

## CONTROL

For the control of toxoplasmosis in goat herds, attention must be paid to the packing of feed, water source and the access of other animals, especially, felids, rodents and birds, to goat house facilities. Such animals may be potential reservoirs of *T. gondii* and other etiologic agents. Therefore, containers intended for drinking water and food must be capped, suspended and housed in places that allow constant cleaning to avoid contamination by different pathogens, including *T. gondii*.

## TREATMENT

Treatment of human toxoplasmosis is not recommended for immunocompetent patients, except for in the early stages of *T. gondii* infection, so it is not recommended for pregnant women, newborns, and immunocompromised patients.

In animals, the therapy protocols are usually applied in abortion outbreak in which there are laboratory confirmations of *T. gondii* infection, and the protocols consist of antibiotics and antiparasitic. Antibiotics correspond to a combination of sulfa drug and trimethoprim, which together have potentiated bacteriostatic actions.

Antiparasitics are administered as prophylactic measures to the pregnant females in order to avoid abortions. Among medicines, monensin and decoquinate may be used, which are usually added to feed.

Monensin, when used as a coccidiostat, forms complexes with sodium and potassium ions inhibiting their transport, substrate oxidation and hydrolysis of adenosine triphosphate (ATP) of trophozoite [46, 47] decoquinate acts at the first stage of life of the protozoan [48].

Existing commercial vaccines for toxoplasmosis are more commonly used in sheep and widely used in countries such as Australia, New Zealand and England [49].

In this chapter, we highlight the importance of vertical transmission by *T. gondii* for both infection and toxoplasmic reinfection, with or without congenital defects, in goats. We elucidate the high dissemination of this zoonosis and the consequent losses in the goatherd resulting from the disposal of positive animals of the property, causing high costs for the breeder. We emphasize on the need to invest in health education to guide the public about consumption of goat products and control of toxoplasmosis in this animal species.

## CONSENT FOR PUBLICATION

Not applicable.

## CONFLICT OF INTEREST

The authors declare no conflict of interest, financial or otherwise.

## ACKNOWLEDGEMENTS

Declared none

## REFERENCES

[1]    Dubey JP. Toxoplasmosis in goats. Agri-prac 1987; 3: 43-52.

[2]    Dubey JP, Adams DS. Prevalence of *Toxoplasma gondii* antibodies in dairy goats from 1982 to 1984. J A Vet Med Assoc 1990; 196: 295-6.

[3]    Cavalcante AC, Carneiro M, Gouveia AM, *et al.* Risk factors for infection by *Toxoplasma gondii* in herds of goats in Ceará, Brazil. Arq Bras Med Vet Zootec 2008; 1: 36-41.
[http://dx.doi.org/10.1590/S0102-09352008000100006]

[4]    Carneiro AC, Carneiro M, Gouveia AM, *et al.* Seroprevalence and risk factors of caprine toxoplasmosis in Minas Gerais, Brazil. Vet Parasitol 2009; 160(3-4): 225-9.
[http://dx.doi.org/10.1016/j.vetpar.2008.10.092] [PMID: 19091475]

[5]    Fredriksson G, Buxton D, Uggla A, *et al.* The effect of *Toxoplasma gondii* infection in unvaccinated and Iscom-vaccinated pregnant ewes as monitored by plasma levels of 15-ketodihydroprostaglandin F2α, progesterone, and oestrone sulphate. J Vet Medic Series A 1990; 1-10: 113-22.

[6]    Vogt Engeland I, Waldeland H, Kindahl H, *et al.* Effect of *Toxoplasma gondii* infection on the development of pregnancy and on endocrine foetal – placental function in the goat. Vet Parasitol 1996; 61: 61-74.
[http://dx.doi.org/10.1016/S0304-4017(96)01025-4] [PMID: 8750684]

[7]    Luft BJ. Toxoplasma gondii. Parasitic Dis Compromised Host. 1989; pp. 179-279.

[8]    Boothroyd JC. *Toxoplasma gondii*: 25 years and 25 major advances for the field. Int J Parasitol 2009; 39(8): 935-46.
[http://dx.doi.org/10.1016/j.ijpara.2009.02.003] [PMID: 19630140]

[9]    da Silva RC, Langoni H. *Toxoplasma gondii*: host-parasite interaction and behavior manipulation. Parasitol Res 2009; 105(4): 893-8.
[http://dx.doi.org/10.1007/s00436-009-1526-6] [PMID: 19548003]

[10]   Esteban-Redondo I, Maley SW, Thomson K, *et al.* Detection of *T. gondii* in tissues of sheep and cattle following oral infection. Vet Parasitol 1999; 86(3): 155-71.

[http://dx.doi.org/10.1016/S0304-4017(99)00138-7] [PMID: 10511098]

[11] Dubey JP. Lesions in transplacentally induced toxoplasmosis in goats. Am J Vet Res 1988; 49(6): 905-9.
[PMID: 3400927]

[12] Montaño PY, Cruz MA, Ullmann LS, *et al.* Contato com gatos: um fator de risco para a toxoplasmose congênita? Clin Vet 2010; 86: 78-84.

[13] Beverley JK, Watson WA, Spence JB. The pathology of the foetus in ovine abortion due to toxoplasmosis. Vet Rec 1971; 88(7): 174-8.
[http://dx.doi.org/10.1136/vr.88.7.174] [PMID: 5102171]

[14] Watson WA, Beverley JK. Epizootics of toxoplasmosis causing ovine abortion. Vet Rec 1971; 88(5): 120-4.
[http://dx.doi.org/10.1136/vr.88.5.120] [PMID: 5547734]

[15] Miller JK, Blewett DA, Buxton D. Clinical and serological response of pregnant gimmers to experimentally induced toxoplasmosis. Vet Rec 1982; 111(6): 124-6.
[http://dx.doi.org/10.1136/vr.111.6.124] [PMID: 7123831]

[16] Blewett DA, Teale AJ, Miller JK, Scott GR, Buxton D. Toxoplasmosis in rams: possible significance of venereal transmission. Vet Rec 1982; 111(4): 73-5.
[http://dx.doi.org/10.1136/vr.111.4.73] [PMID: 6897139]

[17] Silva HM, Pereira MM, Oliveira TA, *et al.* Congenital transmission in reinfected goats with Toxoplasma gondii. Rev Cient Med Vet 2014; pp. 1-21.

[18] Silva HM, Pereira MM, Oliveira TA, *et al.* Goats reinfected with *Toxoplasma gondii*: loss of viable prolificacy and gross revenue. Arq Bras Med Vet Zootec 2015; 67: 1279-86.
[http://dx.doi.org/10.1590/1678-4162-7160]

[19] Vitor RW, Ferreira AM, Fux B. Antibody response in goats experimentally infected with *Toxoplasma gondii.* Vet Parasitol 1999; 81(3): 259-63.
[http://dx.doi.org/10.1016/S0304-4017(98)00251-9] [PMID: 10190869]

[20] Nishi SM, Kasai N, Gennari SM. Antibody levels in goats fed *Toxoplasma gondii* oocysts. J Parasitol 2001; 87(2): 445-7.
[http://dx.doi.org/10.1645/0022-3395(2001)087[0445:ALIGFT]2.0.CO;2] [PMID: 11318584]

[21] Santana LF, da Costa AJ, Pieroni J, *et al.* Detection of *Toxoplasma gondii* in the reproductive system of male goats. Rev Bras Parasitol Vet 2010; 19(3): 179-82.
[http://dx.doi.org/10.1590/S1984-29612010000300010] [PMID: 20943023]

[22] Abouzeid NZ, Amer HA, Barakat TM, *et al.* Toxoplasmosis in naturally and experimentally infected goats. J Am Sci 2010; 6: 122-9.

[23] Dubey JP, Kirkbride CA. Enzootic toxoplasmosis in sheep in north-central United States. J Parasitol 1989; 75(5): 673-6.
[http://dx.doi.org/10.2307/3283047] [PMID: 2795369]

[24] Camargo ME, Silva SM, Leser PG, *et al.* Avidez de anticorpos IgG específicos como marcadores de infecção primária recente pelo *Toxoplasma gondii.* Rev Inst Med Trop 1991; 3: 213-8.
[http://dx.doi.org/10.1590/S0036-46651991000300008]

[25] Vaughan L. Abortion in sheep. Compendium on Continuing Education for the Practicing Veterinary 1996; 3: 170-4.

[26] Wooding FB. Current topic: the synepitheliochorial placenta of ruminants: binucleate cell fusions and hormone production. Placenta 1992; 13(2): 101-13.
[http://dx.doi.org/10.1016/0143-4004(92)90025-O] [PMID: 1631024]

[27] Agerholm JS, Aalbaek B, Fog-Larsen AM, *et al.* Veterinary and medical aspects of abortion in Danish sheep. Act Pathol. Microbiol et Immunol Scan 2006; 2: 146-52.

[28]    Broaddus CC, Lamm CG, Kapil S, Dawson L, Holyoak GR. Bovine viral diarrhea virus abortion in goats housed with persistently infected cattle. Vet Pathol 2009; 46(1): 45-53.
[http://dx.doi.org/10.1354/vp.46-1-45] [PMID: 19112114]

[29]    Marques PX, O'Donovan J, Williams EJ, *et al.* Detection of *Toxoplasma gondii* antigens reactive with antibodies from serum, amniotic, and allantoic fluids from experimentally infected pregnant ewes. Vet Parasitol 2012; 185(2-4): 91-100.
[http://dx.doi.org/10.1016/j.vetpar.2011.10.028] [PMID: 22088616]

[30]    Gutierrez J, O'Donovan J, William E, *et al.* Detection and quantification of *Toxoplasma gondii* in ovine maternal and foetal tissues from experimentally infected pregnant ewes using real-time PCR. Vet Parasitol 2010; 172: 8-15.

[31]    ANVISA – Agência Nacional de Vigilância Sanitária. Resolução RDC N° 216, de 15 de setembro de 2004: Dispõe sobre o Regulamento Técnico de Boas Práticas para Serviços de Alimentação. 2017 Dez 04.. 2017.http://portal.anvisa.gov.br/ documents/33916/ 388704/ RESOLU%25C3% 2587%25C3% 2583O-RDC% 2BN%2B216% 2BDE%2B15% 2BDE%2BSETEMBRO% 2BDE%2B2004.pdf/ 23701496-925d-4d4d-99aa-9d479b316c4b

[32]    IDF - International Dairy Federation e FAO - Food and Agriculture Organization of the United Nations. Guia de boas práticas na pecuária de leite. Produção e Saúde Animal Diretrizes 2013; 8, p. 51.

[33]    Cook AJ, Gilbert RE, Buffolano W, *et al.* Sources of *toxoplasma* infection in pregnant women: European multicentre case-control study. BMJ 2000; 321(7254): 142-7.
[http://dx.doi.org/10.1136/bmj.321.7254.142] [PMID: 10894691]

[34]    Da Silva AV, Langoni H, *et al.* Foods of animal origin and human toxoplasmosis. Hig Aliment 2000; 71: 34-9.

[35]    de Almeida MJ, de Oliveira LH, Freire RL, Navarro IT. Aspectos sociopolíticos da epidemia de toxoplasmose em Santa Isabel do Ivaí (PR). Cien Saude Colet 2011; 16(01) (Suppl. 1): 1363-73.
[http://dx.doi.org/10.1590/S1413-81232011000700071] [PMID: 21503487]

[36]    Renoiner EI, Siqueira AA, Garcia MH, *et al.* 2007.portal.saude.gov.br/ portal/.../ ano07_n08_ toxopl_ adquirida_ go.pdf

[37]    Jones JL, Dargelas V, Roberts J, Press C, Remington JS, Montoya JG. Risk factors for *Toxoplasma gondii* infection in the United States. Clin Infect Dis 2009; 49(6): 878-84.
[http://dx.doi.org/10.1086/605433] [PMID: 19663709]

[38]    de Almeida MJ, de Oliveira LH, Freire RL, Navarro IT. Aspectos sociopolíticos da epidemia de toxoplasmose em Santa Isabel do Ivaí (PR). Cien Saude Colet 2011; 16(1) (Suppl. 1): 1363-73.
[http://dx.doi.org/10.1590/S1413-81232011000700071] [PMID: 21503487]

[39]    Riemann HP, Meyer ME, Theis JH, Kelso G, Behymer DE. Toxoplasmosis in an infant fed unpasteurized goat milk. J Pediatr 1975; 87(4): 573-6.
[http://dx.doi.org/10.1016/S0022-3476(75)80825-0] [PMID: 1171952]

[40]    Dubey JP. Mouse pathogenicity of *Toxoplasma gondii* isolated from a goat. Am J Vet Res 1980; 41(3): 427-9.
[PMID: 7369619]

[41]    Sacks JJ, Roberto RR, Brooks NF. Toxoplasmosis infection associated with raw goat's milk. JAMA 1982; 248(14): 1728-32.
[http://dx.doi.org/10.1001/jama.1982.03330140038029] [PMID: 7120593]

[42]    Chiari CA, Neves DP, Pereira ND. Toxoplasmose humana adquirida através da ingestão de leite de cabra. Mem Inst Oswaldo Cruz 1984; 3: 337-40.
[http://dx.doi.org/10.1590/S0074-02761984000300007]

[43]    Vitor RW, Pinto JB, Chiari CA. Eliminação de *Toxoplasma gondii* através de urina, saliva e leite de

caprinos experimentalmente infectados. Arq Bras Med Vet Zootec 1991; 43: 147-54.

[44]     Dubey JP. Toxoplasmosis. J Am Vet Med Assoc 1994; 205(11): 1593-8.
[PMID: 7730132]

[45]     Pepin M, Russo P, Pardon P. Public health hazards from small ruminant meat products in Europe. Rev Sci Tech off Int Epiz 1997; 16: 415-25.
[http://dx.doi.org/10.20506/rst.16.2.1040]

[46]     Roberson EL. Antiprotozoan drugs.McDonald LM Veterinary pharmacology and therapeutics. 4th ed. Ames: The Iowa State Universaty Press 1978; pp. 1084-5.

[47]     Edds GT, Bortell R. Monensin-Rumensin/ Coban indications and adverse effects. Proceeding of the United States Animal Health Association Aishville 1982; 86: 375-6.

[48]     de Andrade AL Jr, da Silva PC, de Aguiar EM, Santos FG. Use of coccidiostat in mineral salt and study on ovine eimeriosis. Rev Bras Parasitol Vet 2012; 21(1): 16-21.
[http://dx.doi.org/10.1590/S1984-29612012000100004] [PMID: 22534939]

[49]     Porto WJ, Andrade MR. MOTA RA. Toxoplasmose e neosporose em caprinos e ovinos. Ciênc Vet Tróp 2015; 2: 109-12.

# CHAPTER 8

# Congenital Toxoplasmosis in Cattle

**Thaís Rabelo dos Santos[1,*], Maerle Oliveira Maia[2], Jancarlo Ferreira Gomes[3,4], Celso Tetsuo Nagase Suzuki[4], Alvimar José da Costa[5] and Katia Denise Saraiva Bresciani[6]**

[1] *UFVJM, Universidade Federal dos Vales do Jequitinhonha e Mucuri, Instituto de Ciências Agrárias, Unaí, Minas Gerais, Brasil*

[2] *UFMT, Universidade Federal do Mato Grosso, Faculdade de Medicina Veterinária, Cuiabá, Mato Grosso, Brasil*

[3] *UNICAMP, Universidade Estadual de Campinas, Instituto de Biologia, Campinas, São Paulo, Brasil*

[4] *UNICAMP, Universidade Estadual de Campinas, Instituto de Computação, Campinas, São Paulo, Brasil*

[5] *UNESP, Universidade Estadual Paulista (Unesp), Faculdade de Ciências Agrárias e Veterinárias de Jaboticabal, CPPAR, Centro de Pesquisas em Sanidade Animal, Jaboticabal, São Paulo, Brasil*

[6] *UNESP, Universidade Estadual Paulista Júlio de Mesquita Filho, Faculdade de Medicina Veterinária de Araçatuba, Araçatuba, São Paulo, Brasil. Research ID E-7126-2012*

**Abstract:** *Toxoplasma gondii* is a parasite of the phylum Apicomplexa. It is an obligate intracellular protozoan that affects humans and a diverse range of vertebrate hosts. The infection of herbivores occurs primarily through ingestion of oocysts in food and contaminated soils and water. Natural infection by *T. gondii* in cattle was originally reported in Ohio, USA, which also reported the first experimental infection by this protozoan in cattle. The congenital transmission of *T. gondii* in cattle was originally described in 1980. The congenital transmission may frequently be affected by the pathogenicity of the *T. gondii* strain and this zoonotic parasite is example of endogenous and exogenous transplacental infection, which emphasizes the need for greater precision in describing field or experimental research that describes infection passing from cows to fetuses, as well as the actual importance of cattle, in different countries, on the epidemiology of toxoplasmosis.

**Keywords:** Abortion, Bioassay, Cat, Diagnosis, ELISA, Endogenous transplacental infection, Exogenous transplacental infection, IFA, Oocysts, Pathogenicity, PCR, Prevalence, Tachyzoites, *Toxoplasma gondii*, Transmission.

* **Corresponding author Thaís Rabelo dos Santos:** UFVJM, Universidade Federal dos Vales do Jequitinhonha e Mucuri, Instituto de Ciências Agrárias, Unaí, Minas Gerais, Brasil; E-mail: rabelo.vet@hotmail.com

# INTRODUCTION

*Toxoplasma gondii* is a parasite of the phylum *Apicomplexa*. It is an obligate intracellular protozoan [1] that affects humans and many vertebrate hosts [2, 3].

Approximately 30% of the human population has antibodies against this protozoan [10], and the prevalence is even higher in other parts of Europe, Central America and South America [11].

Evaluation of natural occurrence of *T. gondii* antibodies in cattle has drawn the attention of researchers worldwide [3 - 7]. This indicates that new research on bovine toxoplasmosis should be performed, in order to investigate on the actual importance of cattle, in different countries, on the epidemiology of toxoplasmosis [8].

It has been shown that congenital infection of *T. gondii* in cattle, while infrequent, does occur naturally [9]. The pathogenicity of the strain of *T. gondii* may influence the likelihood of this route of transmission.

# EPIDEMIOLOGY

The current literature presents values ranging from zero to 92% regarding the presence of anti-*T.gondii* antibodies in cattle [12]. In Brazil, the seroprevalence has been between 50% and 80%. Some countries, such as Japan, Portugal and Sudan, have low prevalence, *i.e.,* < 20% [13 - 15]. However, Australia, Poland, UK and Belgium show average prevalence (between 23 and 53%), while Tahiti and France have high prevalence (> 60%) [16]. In Brazil, variation in prevalence of values has also been observed, ranging from 1.03% [4] to 71% [4].

A study performed in 1994 concluded that cattle may be relatively resistant to infection, since occurrence of cysts in the muscles is less frequent and persists for shorter time as compared to other animal species [2].

Recent studies in Netherlands demonstrated that seroprevalence cannot be used as an indicator of the number of cattle carrying infectious parasites and suggested that only recent infections are detectable [17]. Serological testing by MAT does not provide information about the presence of *T. gondii* in cattle and does not provide an indication of the risk for consumers [18].

*T. gondii* appears to be less infective to cows at various stages of gestation as compared with ewes and bitches [19]. Using calves inoculated with *T. gondii* oocysts, studies found viable cysts in muscles for up to 1191 days post-infection, but antibody titers remained high for two years, and became serologically negative after this period [20]. Despite the *T. gondii* isolation being more difficult, it can be obtained from bovine retina and diaphragm, and congenital transmission has been confirmed by the presence of the parasite in fetuses of pregnant cows [21].

Some studies found that toxoplasmosis is the third leading cause of foodborne deaths in the United States, and it has been estimated that there are approximately 1.5 million new acute infections per year, with 15% being asymptomatic [22]. It has been reported that the transmission of *T. gondii* by ingestion of oocysts is the most common route of infection in Latin America [23, 24].

In Europe, the percentage of foodborne toxoplasmosis infection is not known, however it has been estimated between 30 and 63% [25]. Direct contact with felines had little epidemiological consequences. However, the presence of infected animals may indicate a contaminated environment, incurring risk to the human population and other animals [7].

## DIAGNOSIS

Confirmation of the diagnosis depends on isolation of the parasite, demonstration of the organism in histological lesions and positive serodiagnosis.

Serological diagnosis can be performed showing ascending titration of anti-*T. gondii* in paired sera or by demonstration of high titer antibody serum in a single serum sample, but lack of ascending or high titration does not exclude the diagnosis of toxoplasmosis [26]. There are several valid serological tests, with the most common ones being the IFA, IHA, complement fixation (CF), and ELISA [27]. The sensitivity and specificity of the rSAG1-ELISA ranged from 67.20 to 94.67% and 71.78 to 96.52%, respectively with respect to IFAT [28].

Previously, there has also been developed the coloring test, also known as the Dye Test [29]. Posteriorly, development of an agglutination test was performed, which revealed low specificity and the need of a large number of tachyzoites in each test [30]. Subsequently, other studies improved reproducibility and sensitivity of the method [31]. There is a wide variation in the prevalence of *T. gondii* infection in different regions of the world due to the different techniques employed, making results not amenable to comparison [32]. The IFA is the most widely used test for diagnosis of toxoplasmosis, which is being used as the gold standard. For this, titers of 16 or higher were considered positive for *T. gondii* [33]. Currently, titers higher or equal to 64 are considered positive [34, 35].

## CONGENITAL TOXOPLASMOSIS

Natural infection by *T. gondii* in cattle was originally reported in Ohio, USA [36], by the same researchers who also reported the first experimental infection by this protozoan in cattle.

Later, studies described the congenital transmission of *T. gondii* in cattle [17 - 19]. While studying *Toxoplasma* infection in experimentally infected gestating cows, these authors isolated *T. gondii* from the brain and liver of four cows, from the placenta of two cows and from the gastric contents of two fetuses. In addition, one cow aborted 24 days after intravenous inoculation with *T. gondii* tachyzoites (strain not reported) [37].

Cattle are susceptible to infection but resistant to disease induced by *T. gondii* [38], rendering them a poor host because, although cattle can be successfully infected with *T. gondii* oocysts, the parasite is eliminated or reduced to undetectable levels within a few weeks [39].

The terms like 'vertical' (transmitted from one generation to the next), 'congenital' (present at birth, acquired in utero or in reproductive cell) and 'transplacental' (acquired in utero) were considered as inadequate for describing the transmission of an infection from one generation to the next [40]. With the relatively recent discovery of *Neospora caninum* and the elucidation of its transmission modes in cattle, together with consideration of the transmission characteristics of the related apicomplexan parasite *T. gondii*, it is apparent that none of the above terms is precise enough to distinguish two extremely different transmission scenarios. These researchers advocate the use of the terms 'endogenous transplacental infection (TPI)' and 'exogenous TPI' to describe, respectively, the TPI of an agent from a pre-existing chronic infection of the dam (which, itself, was probably infected in utero) and a TPI that results from infection of the dam when pregnant.

*T. gondii* was not isolated from the blood of calves and pregnant cows infected with oocysts [20]. Another trial, using the same protocols, was not able to isolate *T. gondii* from zebu cows [41].

In Switzerland, *T. gondii* DNA was detected in 5% of bovine aborted fetuses (n = 2). It demonstrates that *T. gondii* can be transmitted transplacentally in cattle, but it is probably a rare occurrence [41].

In a different experiment, authors infected *Bos taurus*, *Bos indicus*, and *Bubalus bubalis* with *T. gondii* oocysts orally, and described that *B. taurus* were more affected than the other species [43].

Some studies failed to demonstrate *T. gondii* in cattle fetuses [44]. During the course of attempts to isolate, *T. gondii* was isolated from two aborted fetuses, one from Portugal and one from the United States. The isolates were made by bioassay of fetal brains in mice. The fetus from Portugal was about 5 months of gestational age, and the fetus from the United States was a full-term stillborn. Whether *T. gondii* was actually the cause of abortion in the study could not be determined because the brains were not examined histologically. Abortion of cows in the last 12 months was associated with the high rate of seroprevalence for toxoplasmosis [7].

Utilizing one uninfected pregnant heifer as control, and four with *T. gondii* RH strain at their midgestational period, it was observed that the infected group showed clinical signs and antibodies for *T. gondii*, while the control animal was normal [45]. Two (50%) *Toxoplasma* cows were aborted on day 6 and 11 were aborted post inoculation. *T. gondii* tachyzoites were found in various organs of those cows that had abortions but not in their fetuses. The remaining two *Toxoplasma* cows became recumbent. Those two cows and their fetuses showed disseminated *Toxoplasma* DNA. Such findings suggest that maternal toxoplasmosis could be a cause of abortion and congenital toxoplasmosis in cattle, especially when they are infected by virulent strains.

Congenital infection of *T. gondii* in cattle can occur under natural conditions. Regarding the experimental infection of *T. gondii* in pregnant cows, the studies failed to isolate it from any of the nine fetuses born to cows that were experimentally infected with *T. gondii* oocysts. The frequency of congenital transmission may be affected by the pathogenicity of the *T. gondii* strain under study [9]. Then, *T. gondii* can be transmitted transplacentally in cattle [44], but it has not been suggested that this parasite is an important bovine abortifacient [46].

## CONCLUDING REMARKS

Frequently, congenital transmission may be affected by the pathogenicity of the *T. gondii* strain and this zoonotic parasite presents endogenous and exogenous transplacental infection, emphasizing the need for greater precision in describing field or experimental research that describes infection passing from cows to fetuses, as well as the actual importance of cattle, in different countries, on the epidemiology of toxoplasmosis.

## CONSENT FOR PUBLICATION

Not applicable.

## CONFLICT OF INTEREST

The authors declare no conflict of interest, financial or otherwise.

## ACKNOWLEDGEMENTS

Declared none

## REFERENCES

[1]     Rorman E, Zamir CS, Rilkis I, Ben-David H. Congenital toxoplasmosis--prenatal aspects of *Toxoplasma gondii* infection. Reprod Toxicol 2006; 21(4): 458-72.
        [http://dx.doi.org/10.1016/j.reprotox.2005.10.006] [PMID: 16311017]

[2]     Dubey JP. Toxoplasmosis. J Am Vet Med Assoc 1994; 205(11): 1593-8.
        [PMID: 7730132]

[3]     Sharif M, Gholami Sh, Ziaei H, *et al.* Seroprevalence of *Toxoplasma gondii* in cattle, sheep and goats slaughtered for food in Mazandaran province, Iran, during 2005. Vet J 2007; 174(2): 422-4.
        [http://dx.doi.org/10.1016/j.tvjl.2006.07.004] [PMID: 16919980]

[4]     Pita Gondim LF, Barbosa HV Jr, Ribeiro Filho CH, Saeki H. Serological survey of antibodies to *Toxoplasma gondii* in goats, sheep, cattle and water buffaloes in Bahia State, Brazil. Vet Parasitol 1999; 82(4): 273-6.
        [http://dx.doi.org/10.1016/S0304-4017(99)00033-3] [PMID: 10384902]

[5]     Nematollahi A, Moghddam G. Survey on seroprevalence of Anti-*Toxoplasma gondii* antibodies in Cattle in Tabriz Iran by IFAT. Am J Anim Vet Sci 2008; 3: 40-2.
        [http://dx.doi.org/10.3844/ajavsp.2008.40.42]

[6]     Spagnol FH, Paranhos EB, Oliveira LL, de Medeiros SM, Lopes CW, Albuquerque GR. Prevalência de anticorpos anti-*Toxoplasma gondii* em bovinos abatidos em matadouros do estado da Bahia, Brasil. Rev Bras Parasitol Vet 2009; 18(2): 42-5.
        [http://dx.doi.org/10.4322/rbpv.01802009] [PMID: 19602316]

[7]     Santos TR, Costa AJ, Toniollo GH, *et al.* Prevalence of anti-*Toxoplasma gondii* antibodies in dairy cattle, dogs, and humans from the Jauru micro-region, Mato Grosso state, Brazil. Vet Parasitol 2009; 161(3-4): 324-6.
        [http://dx.doi.org/10.1016/j.vetpar.2009.01.017] [PMID: 19232473]

[8]     Dubey JP, Lindsay DS. Neosporosis, toxoplasmosis, and sarcocystosis in ruminants. Vet Clin North Am Food Anim Pract 2006; 22(3): 645-71.
        [http://dx.doi.org/10.1016/j.cvfa.2006.08.001] [PMID: 17071358]

[9]     Costa GH, da Costa AJ, Lopes WD, *et al. Toxoplasma gondii*: infection natural congenital in cattle and an experimental inoculation of gestating cows with oocysts. Exp Parasitol 2011; 127(1): 277-81.
        [http://dx.doi.org/10.1016/j.exppara.2010.08.005] [PMID: 20736009]

[10]    Pena HF, Soares RM, Amaku M, Dubey JP, Gennari SM. *Toxoplasma gondii* infection in cats from São Paulo state, Brazil: seroprevalence, oocyst shedding, isolation in mice, and biologic and molecular characterization. Res Vet Sci 2006; 81(1): 58-67.
        [http://dx.doi.org/10.1016/j.rvsc.2005.09.007] [PMID: 16289158]

[11]    Dubey JP. Strategies to reduce transmission of *Toxoplasma gondii* to animals and humans. Vet Parasitol 1996; 64(1-2): 65-70.
        [http://dx.doi.org/10.1016/0304-4017(96)00961-2] [PMID: 8893464]

[12]    Tenter AM, Heckeroth AR, Weiss LM. *Toxoplasma gondii*: from animals to humans. Int J Parasitol 2000; 30(12-13): 1217-58.
        [http://dx.doi.org/10.1016/S0020-7519(00)00124-7] [PMID: 11113252]

[13]    Matsuo K, Kamai R, Uetsu H, Goto H, Takashima Y, Nagamune K. Seroprevalence of *Toxoplasma gondii* infection in cattle, horses, pigs and chickens in Japan. Parasitol Int 2014; 63(4): 638-9.
[http://dx.doi.org/10.1016/j.parint.2014.04.003] [PMID: 24780140]

[14]    Lopes AP, Dubey JP, Neto F, *et al.* Seroprevalence of *Toxoplasma gondii* infection in cattle, sheep, goats and pigs from the North of Portugal for human consumption. Vet Parasitol 2013; 193(1-3): 266-9.
[http://dx.doi.org/10.1016/j.vetpar.2012.12.001] [PMID: 23290614]

[15]    Medani MY, Kamil IY. Serosurvey of *Toxoplasma gondii* in sheep and cattle for human consumption in Khartoum slaughterhouses, Sudan. Int J Infect Dis 2014; 215: 1-460.

[16]    Avelino MM, Campos D Jr, do Carmo Barbosa de Parada J, de Castro AM. Pregnancy as a risk factor for acute toxoplasmosis seroconversion. Eur J Obstet Gynecol Reprod Biol 2003; 108(1): 19-24.
[http://dx.doi.org/10.1016/S0301-2115(02)00353-6] [PMID: 12694964]

[17]    Opsteegh M, Schares G, Blaga R. Experimental studies of *Toxoplasma gondii* in the main livestock species (GP/EFSA/BIOHAZ/2013/01) Final report. EFSA supporting publication 2016; EN-995: 161 pp.

[18]    Opsteegh M, Teunis P, Züchner L, Koets A, Langelaar M, van der Giessen J. Low predictive value of seroprevalence of *Toxoplasma gondii* in cattle for detection of parasite DNA. Int J Parasitol 2011; 41(3-4): 343-54.
[http://dx.doi.org/10.1016/j.ijpara.2010.10.006] [PMID: 21145321]

[19]    Stalheim OH, Hubbert WT, Boothe AD, *et al.* Experimental toxoplasmosis in calves and pregnant cows. Am J Vet Res 1980; 41(1): 10-3.
[PMID: 7362114]

[20]    Dubey JP, Thulliez P. Persistence of tissue cysts in edible tissues of cattle fed *Toxoplasma gondii* oocysts. Am J Vet Res 1993; 54(2): 270-3.
[PMID: 8430937]

[21]    Amato Neto V, Medeiros EA, Levi GC, Duarte MI. Toxoplasmose. 4th ed. São Paulo: Savier 1995; p. 154.

[22]    Mead PS, Slutsker L, Dietz V, *et al.* Food-related illness and death in the United States Emerging Infectious Diseases 1999; 5: 607-25.

[23]    Giraldi N, Vidotto O, Navarro IT, Garcia JL, Ogawa L, Kobylka E. Toxoplasma antibody and stool parasites in public school children, Rolândia, Paraná, Brazil. Rev Soc Bras Med Trop 2002; 35(3): 215-9.
[http://dx.doi.org/10.1590/S0037-86822002000300003] [PMID: 12045813]

[24]    Santos SL, de Souza Costa K, Gondim LQ, *et al.* Investigation of *Neospora caninum, Hammondia sp.*, and *Toxoplasma gondii* in tissues from slaughtered beef cattle in Bahia, Brazil. Parasitol Res 2010; 106(2): 457-61.
[http://dx.doi.org/10.1007/s00436-009-1686-4] [PMID: 19943064]

[25]    van der Giessen J, Fonville M, Bouwknegt M, Langelaar M, Vollema A. Seroprevalence of Trichinella spiralis and *Toxoplasma gondii* in pigs from different housing systems in The Netherlands. Vet Parasitol 2007; 148(3-4): 371-4.
[http://dx.doi.org/10.1016/j.vetpar.2007.06.009] [PMID: 17646053]

[26]    Lappin MR. Infecções protozoárias e mistas. 2004.

[27]    Sikes RK. Toxoplasmosis. J Am Vet Med Assoc 1982; 180(8): 857-9.
[PMID: 7085463]

[28]    Sudan V, Tewari AK, Singh H. Serodiagnosis of *Toxoplasma gondii* infection in bovines from Kerala, India using a recombinant surface antigen 1 ELISA. Biologicals 2015; 43(4): 250-5.
[http://dx.doi.org/10.1016/j.biologicals.2015.04.002] [PMID: 25952097]

[29] Sabin AB, Feldman HA. Dyes as microchemical indicators of a rew immunity phenomenon affecting a protozoon parasite (Toxoplasma). Science 1948; 108(2815): 660-3.
[http://dx.doi.org/10.1126/science.108.2815.660] [PMID: 17744024]

[30] Fulton JD, Turk JL. Direct agglutination test for *Toxoplasma gondii*. Lancet 1959; 2(7111): 1068-9.
[http://dx.doi.org/10.1016/S0140-6736(59)91535-1] [PMID: 13825641]

[31] Desmonts G, Remington JS. Direct agglutination test for diagnosis of Toxoplasma infection: method for increasing sensitivity and specificity. J Clin Microbiol 1980; 11(6): 562-8.
[PMID: 7000807]

[32] Chhabra MB, Gupta SL, Gautam OP. Toxoplasma seroprevalence in animals in northern India. Int J Zoonoses 1985; 12(2): 136-42.
[PMID: 4077411]

[33] Dubey JP, Beattie CP. Toxoplasmosis of animals and man. Boca Raton: CRC Press; 1988. pp. 1-220.

[34] Costa AJ, Araújo FG, Costa JO, Lima JD, Nascimento E. Experimental infection of bovines with oocysts of *Toxoplasma gondii*. J Parasitol 1977; 63(2): 212-8.
[http://dx.doi.org/10.2307/3280042] [PMID: 558305]

[35] Souza LM. Neosporose e toxoplasmose bubaline: estudo da situação sorológica em rebanhos leiteiros do Estado de São Paulo 2001 69f Dissertação (Mestrado em Medicina Veterinária)- Faculdade de Ciências Agrárias e Veterinárias, Universidade Estadual Paulista. Jabotical 2001.

[36] Sanger VL, Chamberlain DM, Chamberlain KW, Cole CR, Farrell RL. Toxoplasmosis. V. Isolation of Toxoplasma from cattle. J Am Vet Med Assoc 1953; 123(917): 87-91.
[PMID: 13069361]

[37] Jungersen G, Bille-Hansen V, Jensen L, Lind P. Transplacental transmission of *Toxoplasma gondii* in minipigs infected with strains of different virulence. J Parasitol 2001; 87(1): 108-13.
[http://dx.doi.org/10.1645/0022-3395(2001)087[0108:TTOTGI]2.0.CO;2] [PMID: 11227873]

[38] Esteban-Redondo I, Innes EA. *Toxoplasma gondii* infection in sheep and cattle. Comp Immunol Microbiol Infect Dis 1997; 20(2): 191-6.
[http://dx.doi.org/10.1016/S0147-9571(96)00039-2] [PMID: 9208205]

[39] Dubey JP, Jones JL. *Toxoplasma gondii* infection in humans and animals in the United States. Int J Parasitol 2008; 38(11): 1257-78.
[http://dx.doi.org/10.1016/j.ijpara.2008.03.007] [PMID: 18508057]

[40] Trees AJ, Williams DJ. Endogenous and exogenous transplacental infection in *Neospora caninum* and *Toxoplasma gondii*. Trends Parasitol 2005; 21(12): 558-61.
[http://dx.doi.org/10.1016/j.pt.2005.09.005] [PMID: 16223599]

[41] Marques FA. Transmissão vertical do Neospora caninum em fêmeas de corte (Bos indicus) abatidas em frigorífico / Francisco Augusto Coelho Marques - Londrina 2009 81f Tese (Doutorado). Londrina: Universidade Estadual de Londrina 2009.

[42] Gottstein B, Hentrich B, Wyss R, *et al*. Molecular and immunodiagnostic investigations on bovine neosporosis in Switzerland. Int J Parasitol 1998; 28(4): 679-91.
[http://dx.doi.org/10.1016/S0020-7519(98)00006-X] [PMID: 9602392]

[43] Oliveira FC, Costa AJ, Sabatini GA. Clínica e hematologia de *Bos indicus, Bos taurus*, e *Bubalus bubalis* inoculados com oocistos de *Toxoplasma gondii* (Apicomplexa: Toxoplasmatinae). Cienc Rural 2001; 31: 621-6.
[http://dx.doi.org/10.1590/S0103-84782001000400010]

[44] Canada N, Meireles CS, Rocha A, da Costa JM, Erickson MW, Dubey JP. Isolation of viable *Toxoplasma gondii* from naturally infected aborted bovine fetuses. J Parasitol 2002; 88(6): 1247-8.
[http://dx.doi.org/10.1645/0022-3395(2002)088[1247:IOVTGF]2.0.CO;2] [PMID: 12537120]

[45] Wiengcharoen J, Thompson RC, Nakthong C, Rattanakorn P, Sukthana Y. Transplacental transmission

in cattle: 1s *Toxoplasma gondii* less potent than Neospora caninum? Parasitol Res 2011; 108(5): 1235-41.
[http://dx.doi.org/10.1007/s00436-010-2172-8] [PMID: 21203773]

[46]     de Macedo MF, de Macedo CA, Ewald MP, *et al.* Isolation and genotyping of *Toxoplasma gondii* from pregnant dairy cows (Bos taurus) slaughtered. Rev Bras Parasitol Vet 2012; 21(1): 74-7.
[http://dx.doi.org/10.1590/S1984-29612012000100016] [PMID: 22534951]

# SUBJECT INDEX

## A

Abortion and stillbirths 71, 97
Acquired toxoplasmosis 37, 42, 62
　congenital 62
Acute infection 5, 23, 24, 28, 42
Acute toxoplasmosis 13, 23, 27, 28, 36, 37, 98
Adverse effects 25, 36, 40, 44
Aminotransferases 36, 45
Amniocentesis 17, 25, 27, 29
Amniotic fluid 25, 63
Anorexia 71, 82, 85, 86, 87
Antibodies 1, 5, 6, 15, 20, 22, 23, 24, 34, 37,
　　38, 63, 67, 71, 75, 77, 79, 82, 83, 84, 87,
　　88, 96, 98, 99, 106, 109
　anti-T.gondii 6, 83, 106
　detecting 87
　detection of 24, 88
　maternal 38, 99
Antibodies anti-*T. gondii* 1
Apicomplexa 1, 2, 61, 82, 105, 106, 108
Aqueous humor 70, 71
Audiometric evaluation 46

## B

Bovines 6
Bradyzoites 1, 2, 3, 4, 68, 76, 88

## C

Caprines 6, 96, 97
Cattle, *T. gondii* 105, 106, 108, 109
Central nervous system (CNS) 39, 67, 68, 69,
　97
Cerebral calcifications 4, 15, 17, 40, 41
Cerebrospinal fluid 39, 41, 44, 71
Chorioretinitis 67, 70, 85
Chronic infections, pre-existing 108
Clindamycin 44, 64, 71
CNS infections 40
Coccidian parasite 1

Coccidium 68
Cohort study 30, 38, 40
Computerized tomography 45, 46
Conducted parasite's DNA 70
Confirmed acute toxoplasmosis 28
Confirmed cases of CT 14, 40
Congenital diseases 75, 76, 78
Congenital forms 68, 69
Congenital infection 1, 4, 17, 18, 22, 23, 30,
　　37, 38, 46, 62, 68, 82, 84, 106, 109
Congenital problems 96
Congenital toxoplasma infections 67
Congenital transmission 4, 19, 62, 77, 78, 79,
　　105, 107, 108, 109
Contaminated food 75, 76
Cyst-forming coccidium *Toxoplasma gondii*
　76

## D

Daraprim 36, 42, 43
Days post-gestation 98
Definitive hosts 3, 7, 19, 67
Detection of IgM antibodies 22, 37
Development 3, 4, 7, 19, 26, 31, 62, 68, 69,
　　107
　fetal 69
Diagnosed sheep abortion 78
Diagnosis 25, 26, 27, 29, 30, 47
　confirmed 25, 27, 47
　direct 87
　fetal 25, 27, 29
　prenatal 25, 26, 27, 29, 30
Diagnosis of CT 37, 38, 39
Diagnostic methods 24, 26, 39
Differences 5, 22, 25, 30, 83, 84, 85, 87
　genetic 85
Differential diagnosis 5, 39
Difficulties 13, 23, 24, 29, 38
Digestion process 3